Janice A. Noack

D1444233

Concept Formalization in Nursing
PROCESS AND PRODUCT

Concept Formalization in Nursing
PROCESS AND PRODUCT

Second Edition

BY THE NURSING DEVELOPMENT CONFERENCE GROUP

Edited by

Dorothea E. Orem, R.N., M.S.N. Ed.
Chairman

RT
84.5
.N86
1979
c.4

SAINT LOUIS UNIVERSITY
SCHOOL OF NURSING
3525 CAROLINE STREET
ST. LOUIS, MISSOURI 63104

Little, Brown and Company, Boston

Copyright © 1979 by Little, Brown and Company (Inc.)

Second Edition

Previous edition copyright © 1973 by Little, Brown and Company (Inc.)

All rights reserved. No part of this book may be reproduced in any form
or by any electronic or mechanical means, including information
storage and retrieval systems, without permission in writing from the
publisher, except by a reviewer who may quote brief passages in a
review.

Library of Congress Catalog Card No. 79-88164

ISBN 0-316-61421-1

Printed in the United States of America

MV

*To Joan E. Backscheider, R.N., Ph.D.,
and Mary B. Collins, R.N., M.S.N.*

Contributing Authors

Dorothea E. Orem, R.N., M.S.N.Ed.
Consultant, Nursing and Nursing Education, Orem and Shields, Inc., Chevy Chase, Maryland; Chairman, Nursing Development Conference Group 1968—1978

PARTICIPATING NURSING DEVELOPMENT CONFERENCE GROUP MEMBERS

Sarah E. Allison, R.N., Ed.D.
Associate Vice-President, Nursing Administration, Mississippi Methodist Hospital and Rehabilitation Center, Jackson, Mississippi

Cora S. Balmat, R.N., Ph.D.
Professor, Graduate Program, School of Nursing, University of Southern Mississippi, Hattiesburg, Mississippi

Judy Crews, R.N., M.S.N.
Cardiovascular Nursing Specialist, Outpatient Nursing Services, The Johns Hopkins Hospital, Baltimore, Maryland

Melba Anger Malatesta, R.N., M.S.N.
Assistant Professor, Division of Nursing, Coppin State College, Baltimore, Maryland

Sheila M. McCarthy, R.N., M.S.N.
Director of Nursing, George Washington University Medical Center, Washington, D.C.

Louise Hartnett Rauckhorst, R.N., M.S.N.
Associate Professor, Boston College School of Nursing, Chestnut Hill, Massachusetts

CONTRIBUTING AUTHORS TO THE FIRST EDITION
*Sarah E. Allison, Joan E. Backscheider, Cora S. Balmat,
Mary B. Collins, M. Lucille Kinlein, Janina B. Lapniewska,
Sheila M. McCarthy, Joan Nettleton, Dorothea E. Orem,
Louise Hartnett Rauckhorst, Helen A. St. Denis*

Preface

In 1968 eleven nurses of varying backgrounds formed the Nursing Development Conference Group. The members of the Group were specialized in particular areas of nursing with experience in nursing practice, teaching, and administration of nursing services and nursing education. The formation and work of the Group were related to members' dissatisfactions with and concerns for the development of nursing as a discipline. The absence of an organizing framework for nursing knowledge and the Group's conviction that the use of a general concept of nursing would aid in formalizing such a framework provided the base for action.

The first edition of *Concept Formalization in Nursing: Process and Product* (1973) represented the initial work of the Group in identifying and describing the conceptual structure of nursing. This 1973 book was a culmination of earlier work initiated in 1965 by the Nursing Model Committee of the Nursing Faculty of The Catholic University of America. Five members of the Conference Group had functioned on this committee, one as chairman, four as committee members.

The second edition of *Concept Formalization in Nursing: Process and Product* includes further developments of the conceptual structure of nursing introduced in the first edition as well as descriptions of the individual and group dynamics associated with formulation, expression, and acceptance of nursing's conceptual structure. The second edition is developed in two parts.

Part I is designed as an orientation to nursing knowledge with a new chapter that is explanatory of nursing's placement in the world of man and human affairs. Part I, with its focus on nursing as a practice discipline, is brought to completion with presentations of selected concepts of nursing in the public domain.

Part II presents the work of the Nursing Development Conference Group with respect to the structure of nursing knowledge. The chapters from the first edition on the concept of nursing system and the dynamics of concept development are included, and some new material has been added. Two new chapters represent a depth development of the nursing system variable "self-care agency." The final chapter brings together the work of individual Group members organized from the perspective of the relation of nursing knowledge to nursing practice.

The composition of the Nursing Development Conference Group has changed with time. The Conference Group members who participated in planning the second edition of the book and who contributed to the work of its development or review have done so with awareness of the nursing contributions of, and the sound foundations for productive group functioning set by, the original eleven. Without these foundations, neither the first nor the second editions could have been written.

The authors express appreciation to nursing students and nurses who have used the book and who have conveyed their constructive ideas to us. Our thinking has been stimulated and advanced in discussions with nurses who have participated with us in seminars and conferences about the structuring of nursing knowledge. The second edition is viewed as a means to promote continued efforts toward the development of nursing sciences.

S. E. A.
C. S. B.
D. E. O.

Contents

Orientations

Nursing Knowledge

The object of this book is to present to the nursing community the ideas of one group of nurses, the Nursing Development Conference Group (hereafter referred to as the NDCG). The NDCG is concerned specifically about the need for and the problems associated with the organization and continuing development of authoritative knowledge about (1) the realities that nurses observe and regulate as nurses and (2) how nurses can effectively observe and regulate these realities.

PRESUPPOSITIONS

The ideas that will be presented rest on the presupposition that nursing as a discipline of authoritative knowledge with patterned meaning [1] is the product of the work of nurses, especially nurses who are scholars, theorists, researchers, and developers. Nurses filling these nursing roles may also be practitioners and teachers. Furthermore, authoritative knowledge[1] is accepted as the element that is created and used by nurses who fulfill role responsibilities in some combination of the five work areas of nursing (i.e., nursing practice, theory development, research, development, and teaching). Effective work in all of these areas is essential for the growth, development, and survival of nursing. Figure 1-1 expresses the idea of the centrality of nursing knowledge; shows articulations among the essential roles of nurses within their field of endeavor, nursing; and suggests role combinations, for example, teacher-scholar or scholar-theorist.

The book is developed from the perspective that nurses engaged in nursing practice know nursing and do nursing and that their knowing nursing is incorporated with their art. The art of nursing is individual and is grounded in those qualities

---

[1]Authoritative knowledge is defined as knowledge that has been formulated and tested by mature nursing scholars functioning in collaboration as members of the discipline nursing.

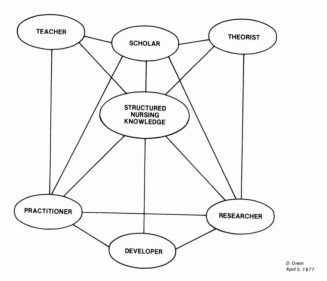

Figure 1-1 Centrality of nursing knowledge in relationship to nurse roles.

of individual nurses that enable them to identify and compose significant elements in themselves and in persons under care in such a way that nursing is created for these persons. Nursing is a product of the nurse's art; it is a human service. Nurses, therefore, must know themselves and those under their care and the relationships between them; nurses must create care and, in so doing, perform specific actions; and before the performance of specific actions, nurses must make choices and decisions about what *can* and what *should* be done.

PRACTICE DISCIPLINES

The generalized and the specific knowledge of nurses that enables them to think nursing and create nursing in accord with their choices and decisions would constitute their psychologically structured nursing knowledge. From this perspective nursing knowledge, when formalized and expressed in the form of laws, theories, concepts, categories of facts, and rules and technologies of practice, would have the form of a *practice discipline*.

Discipline is used in the sense of a scholarly discipline [1, p. 312]. This means an organized field of inquiry in which specialists create or generate authoritative knowledge about entities or things considered from a specific aspect or point of view [1, pp. 95, 101]. *Practice* as a qualifier of discipline means that the generated knowledge is used in the regular performance of a particular kind of work, for example, nursing.

Practice disciplines can be understood in terms of the *knowing, making,* and *doing* orientations of persons engaged in practical endeavors such as the practice of nursing or medicine or engineering. These orientations are represented in Figure 1-2 as interactive aspects of nurse functioning in nursing practice situations. Implicit in the representation is the idea that creating the design for and the making of nursing care (the nurse's art), involving the doing of numerous and specific right actions consequent to the making of prudential judgments and decisions (morals), is informed by the nurse's knowledge of *nursing and related sciences* [1, p. 142]. From the perspective of the nurse there should be continuing awareness[2] of the relationship between the nurse's knowing and doing [2].

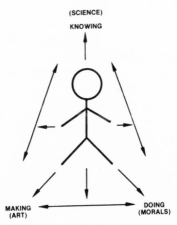

Figure 1-2   Interactive operations of persons engaged in practical endeavors.

[2]This type of awareness is named *rational self-consciousness* by B. J. F. Lonergan [2].

What then are the characteristics of the knowing operations of nurses, and what are the qualities that sciences of nursing would have? Philosophers who write about knowledge in relation to practical endeavors identify it as *derivative or applied* as contrasted with knowledge in *pure or fundamental fields* [1, pp. 272–273, 318–319].

Some philosophers of science suggest that the sciences specific to fields of practical endeavor are of two types — applied sciences and practical sciences. Applied nursing sciences would have as their object the realities that nurses observe and regulate as nurses investigating them from the perspective of nursing and one or more fundamental fields (e.g., physiology or psychology), which yield points of theory explanatory of nursing problems or nursing phenomena. The results of inquiry would be expressed as theories, laws, hypotheses, propositions, general concepts, and as classes and categories of empirical information. Knowledge in the applied nursing sciences would be speculative and explanatory in form, and it affords understanding of the human and environmental factors and conditions significant in nursing practice [3]. Practical nursing science would have as its field of inquiry how nursing can be provided and how nurses can and should regulate their actions under a variety of human and environmental conditions. Practical nursing sciences set forth and provide rationales to guide nursing practice. These include rules, technologies, and the techniques of nursing practice. The practical nursing sciences are thus regulative or normative sciences [3, pp. 314–315].

When developed, the applied nursing sciences would be aids to nurses in understanding the realities, the phenomena upon which nurses focus as nurses, for example, the condition of complete helplessness characteristic of one class of persons who can be helped through nursing. Practical nursing sciences would proceed from the position that, given an existent reality (a person in a state of coma), which the nurse recognizes and understands, then practice should be guided by certain rules, and certain technologies and techniques would have validity under the existent conditions. For the given example, rules of nursing practice would include the rule: *In nursing persons who are comatose, the nurse first acts to facilitate and insure a continuing intake of air.*

Practice disciplines thus are constituted of two kinds of authoritative knowledge. One kind is descriptive and explanatory of nursing realities — the applied nursing sciences. The other kind, practical nursing science, specifies prudential rules [4] to guide the decisions and actions of nurses given specific reality conditions and the preferred technologies and techniques of practice.

THE SITUATION IN NURSING

The more concrete aspects of nursing (i.e., the tasks, including the measures of care that nurses perform) have satisfied and continue to satisfy some nurses as an adequate and appropriate laying out of the domain of nursing practice. Descriptions of these tasks have served nurses as a more or less adequate body of nursing knowledge. However, with the continuing emphasis on the functioning of nurses in empirical inquiry and assessment, and in designing and planning nursing care, the inadequacies of defining and describing nursing in terms of tasks and procedures have become increasingly evident. Nurses can neither attend to nor fulfill responsibilities associated with these operations unless they have (1) rationales that justify what they do as nurses, at the same time being provided with a basis for appraisal and criticism of what they do; (2) descriptive and explanatory knowledge about the realities they observe and regulate as nurses; and (3) knowledge of the rules, technologies, and techniques of practice that are generally applicable or applicable to types of nursing cases.

Nurses, by virtue of their qualifications, represent themselves in society as being able to help others through the provision of nursing. Ideally, nurses direct their attention and effort to human problems that can be solved or mitigated through nursing as distinguished from problems that cannot be so solved or mitigated. This rationale necessitates that nurses know what nursing is designed to do in society in relation to the human conditions that give rise to requirements for it. An adequate nursing rationale that holds for all nursing situations sets forth the reasons for the existence of nursing in societies and provides nurses with criterion measures for distinguishing nursing problems from other human problems.

Nurses who are motivated by the desire to *help others* must know in a general way (in a way applicable to persons in all or some nursing situations) the following:

1. What gives rise to requirements for nursing
2. Types of requirements for nursing
3. Methodologies for identifying care requirements and providing care
4. Rules to guide the decisions and actions of nurses

However, general knowledge is not sufficient in specific situations where nurses provide nursing for individuals or groups. Here nurses must obtain "decisive evidence" through observation of individuals or groups under their care (i.e., evidence enabling them to make judgments about whether there is evidence of presenting requirements for nursing and the specific characteristics of the presenting requirements). When the evidence is inadequate for making such judgments, this needs to be recognized and observation continued.

Thus, in nursing practice there is a requirement that nurses have generalizable nursing knowledge in order to obtain, interpret, and understand the meaning of empirical information about persons or groups under nursing care. The availability of and the form of valid generalizations significant for nursing practice as well as compilations of factual information about persons or groups with specific types of nursing requirements is of critical importance in both practice and educational situations. Mature nursing scholars, theorists, and researchers have special role responsibilities for the availability and the logical structure of nursing knowledge [5]. Nursing knowledge is the product of the specialized endeavors of individual nurses working alone or in collaboration with colleagues. The work of nurses who are nursing scholars, researchers, developers, and theorists is of critical importance to the survival of nursing in a way that will be of future benefit to society.

BASIC AGREEMENTS

Since the beginning of modern nursing, some nurses have been in the forefront of preventive health care. Nurses' understandings of the dimensions of health-care problems often exceed those of colleagues from other disciplines. For these and other reasons the nurse is in an advantageous position to move for constructive change in the expanding field of health services. Far too often, however, too many nurses are inarticulate or unable to speak of nursing in terms that convey the connotation of nursing phenomena, and are unable to describe and represent to others the health-care and health-service problems that are essentially nursing problems. Is not this lack of ability on the part of nurses to participate in a communication process in which nursing content is brought to bear in exploring or solving health-care and service problems due at least in part to the absence of structured nursing knowledge available for use in health-care situations? It may be consoling to say, "Nursing is what nurses do," to get us past the impasse posed by the question, "What is nursing?" However, if there is no concerted effort to describe the reality of, and the bases for, what nurses do, and to generalize from this, nurses will fail to answer the first and essential question in the development of a practice discipline, "What is the case?" much less the more advanced questions, "What can be?" "What should be?"

The nurses whose views are expressed in this book on the basis of their use of a general theory of nursing in the formulation, expression, and application of their understandings of nursing suggest a number of presuppositions that are basic to the psychologic and logical structuring of nursing knowledge.

1. The reliability, validity, and dynamism of nurses' general concepts of what nursing is affects the quality of (a) their nursing practice and (b) the substantive nursing knowledge that will be forthcoming as a result of their efforts to acquire and structure nursing knowledge.
2. Persons prepared through formal education in universities to function as nurses in society ideally view themselves as having role sets related to
   a. Designing, providing, and controlling the quality and quantity of nursing in a society.
   b. Making contributions to the continuing development and refinement of the substantive and syntactical structure of nursing knowledge utilizing appropriate research methodologies.
3. Demands on nursing education in a society arise from
   a. Conditions of nursing practice related to social, cultural, and economic factors that affect it.
   b. The state of development and organization of nursing knowledge and its availability to nursing students and practitioners.
   c. The state of development of nursing-related arts and sciences and the formalization of their articulations with nursing elements.
4. Ideally in the nursing community, role sets of nurses experienced in nursing practice, nursing research, nursing education, or combinations thereof provide for linkages with role sets of neophyte nurses defined in accord with their education and career interests and aspirations. The guidance and supervision provided by experienced nurses are adjusted to both the neophyte status and talents of the nurses to whom they are related.
5. Essential conditions for effective nursing education include the conditions that
   a. Educators have conceptualizations of nursing as a health-care service and as a practice discipline.
   b. Educators be articulate about the elements of each of the above-named concepts and their real-world referents and be able to guide students toward concept formalization and use.

THE PROBLEM

Ideally in a society, there are nurses whose psychologic structuring of nursing knowledge is in advanced states of development. If these nurses guide and direct other nurses who are in less advanced states of knowledge structuring, and consistently contribute to the organization, refinement, and development of a written compendium of nursing knowledge, structured nursing knowledge becomes available within the nursing community.

Professional and technical education in nursing are lengthy exercises in mastering the whole or portions of structured knowledge from a number of diverse but related bodies of knowledge and in using and adding to this knowledge in real-world situations. The paucity of structured knowledge in nursing is becoming increasingly evident to undergraduate and graduate nursing students in college and university nursing programs. Prior and current learning experiences in fields where knowledge is structured provide bases for nursing students' expectations about nursing knowledge within programs of nursing education.

The existence of a logically integrated body of nursing knowledge is often assumed by curriculum workers and nursing planners and developers. Persons in such roles often feel defeated and overwhelmed when confronted by the scope and diversity of the knowledge requirements for effective nursing and the unorganized state of available nursing knowledge. In fact, any in-depth approach to the advancement of nursing practice or curriculum designing demands that the structuring of nursing knowledge become an integral, and at times a principal, part of such projects.

Contemporary nursing practitioners and teachers are confronted not only with the problem of the relatively unstructured state of available nursing knowledge but also with the ever-increasing fund of knowledge within nursing-related disciplines. The task of bringing this knowledge into relationships with elements of nursing is in itself of monumental proportions. Furthermore, it is a task that demands the use of a valid, reliable, and dynamic general concept of what nursing is. How knowledge from other disciplines is to be brought into relationships with nursing knowledge is a matter that demands concerted attention from those members of the nursing community whose psychologic structuring of nursing knowledge is in advanced states of development.

Lack of structure and unclear directions about how to move toward the structuring of nursing knowledge were motivating forces in bringing together the nurses whose ideas and modes of functioning are described and discussed in this and subsequent chapters.

THE GROUP

The NDCG was formed to further a common interest of its members [6]. Members of the NDCG have been engaged in scholarly discourse since September 6, 1968, the date of its initial meeting. At that time it was agreed that the Group would be composed of professional nurses interested in the formalization of theory related to the processes of nursing, with a focus on nursing care. It was recognized that the accomplishment of this purpose demanded that innovations function at the scientific level of nursing practice and that the NDCG afford opportunities for Group members to channel information and structured nursing knowledge for use at the technologic and technical levels of practice [7].

At the time of the inception of the Group, all members filled positions in large organizations — medical center hospitals, university schools of nursing, and a community health agency associated with a university. The experiential nursing backgrounds of members included positions in nursing practice, nursing education, nursing research and development, and the administration thereof. All members are or have been nursing practitioners and all have taught in schools of nursing.

The NDCG is a small, formal organization that has achieved to some degree the characteristics of a true community — fundamental equality, mutual enrichment, membership based on personal interests, and integration of members through personal exchange in accord with talents, abilities, and interests [8]. Specifically, in relation to nursing, the Group is bound together by the commitment of its members to increase the understanding of nursing, including the order that should, can, and sometimes does exist in nursing situations. In this sense, the NDCG is a segment of the larger community of nurses who are concerned with the "gaining of meaning" as described by King and Brownell [9].

Members come together for periods of formal discourse lasting from one to three days. In periods between scheduled Group conferences, members work individually or meet in small work groups related to projects in process. Discourse has contributed not only to furthering the Group interest, but also has increased the productivity of individual members in their various professional roles. Both types of effort, group and individual, are viewed as essential in concept formalization and model development in the movement toward knowledge structuring and discipline development.

A network of professional relationships among members and associates of members has developed during the period of the Group's existence. Forums external to the NDCG have been utilized by members for presentation and discussion of their ideas about nursing. Such extended opportunities are important both in relation to individual and group effort in the determination of the reliability and validity of concepts being utilized in nursing practice and education, and in theory development and research.

Five of the original eleven members of the NDCG were members of its precursor, the Nursing Model Committee of the School of Nursing, The Catholic University of America, Washington, D.C. This committee was initially organized as a subcommittee of the Graduate Curriculum Committee of the School of Nursing for the purpose of developing a model that would express the foundations for, and characteristics of, research in nursing. The members of the Faculty of Nursing who promoted and initiated the formation of the Nursing Model Committee with the assistance of Dean Mary E. Redmond were concerned with the lack of specification of, and agreement about, the general elements of nursing that give direction to (1) the isolation of problems that are specifically nursing problems and (2) the organization of knowledge accruing from research in problem areas.

The Nursing Model Committee functioned effectively from April, 1965, to May, 1968, with a core of stable members as well as a changing membership since the committee was open to all interested members of the faculty. Members included clinical nursing specialists, nursing generalists, and specialists in community-health nursing. The varied nature of the nursing backgrounds of the members was an essential ingredient of the approaches utilized by the committee in arriving at tentative generalizations about nursing. These generalizations were subjected to review and testing by various committee members, some of whom utilized the generalizations in the various curriculum committees on which they functioned.

The Nursing Model Committee presented its final report to the Faculty of the School of Nursing in May, 1968. All committee proceedings and reports, including the listing of members for the years of the committee's existence, were filed in the School of Nursing.

THE NEED AS PERCEIVED BY THE NDCG

The strength of nursing in a society does not rest in the number of nurses or in the number of members of that society who are willing to support nursing at a particular time. The strength of nursing rests in the ability of nurses to tolerate the strain of initiating and keeping preferred nursing systems operational in multiple environments, at the same time deriving satisfaction from their effective actions and from the support received from nursing and other colleagues and from health-care and educational administrators. Since what is preferred varies with the total situation of the individual or group, the preferred system in each nursing situation must be discovered. Knowing the courses of action that are open and estimating the advantages and disadvantages of each in relation to reality factors are aspects of discovery and so provide a basis for decisions and subsequent result-achieving actions of nurses. Structured knowledge enables nurses to bridge the gap between themselves and the external realities of nursing situations and, in so doing, to be in a position to acquire relevant information and in some instances to add to, refine, or restructure knowledge.

Nursing, like other areas of human endeavor, is frequently immersed in problems of the individuals' conflicting goals and in problems arising from prejudice, indifference, and self-interest on the part of nurses and significant others. The maturity of the nurse is a crucial factor in effective practice, teaching, and research. *Personal maturity* is associated with *self-esteem as related to nursing status and role,* which in turn is associated with a *conceptualized and structured body of nursing knowledge* that the individual nurse can utilize. It is the nurse's psychologically structured body of nursing knowledge that provides the basis for *thinking nursing* and safeguards feelings of worth and self-esteem in nurse roles. Thinking nursing means that what nurses perceive in real-world nursing situations is afforded logical meaningfulness by the structured nursing knowledge they already possess or which is made available to them by more knowledgeable nurses. Such knowledge not only affords a nursing significance to what is perceived, but also provides intellectual tools to guide the nurse in assessing the adequacy, validity, and relia-bility of empirical data; it further provides rules and prin-ciples to guide subsequent decision-making and result-achiev-ing activities.

Persons with the status of nurse achieved through formal education ideally are *permitted, expected, able,* and, more-over, *want to think and act as nurses* in real-world nursing situations; they do not want to react merely on the basis of some developed set of habits.

The view of *nurse as reactor* to persons, objects, events, or symbols that they see, hear, or otherwise experience in nurs-ing situations is held by some persons (with or without awareness) within and outside of nursing. The view of nurse as *faithful follower of specific externally imposed rules* set by nursing administrators or physicians or institutional ad-ministrators is in discord with reality demands in nursing situations, behavioral expectations, and sanctions set by law and legal precedent.

Thinking nursing is appropriate nurse behavior; total de-pendence on *action patterns based on habit* is inappropriate behavior for nurses who have benefitted from either pro-fessional or technical forms of education for nursing practice.

Nursing process, nursing judgments, and *nursing decisions* are terms in contemporary nursing literature that imply thinking behaviors based on nursing rules and principles set forth within the framework of a body of knowledge. Nursing elements within the body of knowledge should reflect the real world of nurses and nursing, and bear relationships one to the other and to elements from related bodies of knowledge. As such a body of knowledge becomes increasingly available to nursing students, learning nursing should take on added meaningfulness and economy.

REFERENCES

1. Phenix, P. H.   *Realms of Meaning.* New York: McGraw-Hill, 1964. Pp. 312—313.
2. Lonergan, B. J. F.   *Insight.* New York: Philosophical Library, 1958. Pp. 612—616.
3. Maritain, J. M.   *The Degrees of Knowledge.* New York: Scribner's, 1959. Pp. 311—316, 456—459.
4. Black, M.   *Models and Metaphors.* Ithaca, N.Y.: Cornell University Press. Pp. 95—136.
5. Ausubel, D. P.   Some Psychological Aspects of the Structure of Knowledge. In the *Fifth Annual Phi Delta Kappa Symposium on Educational Research.* Chicago: Rand McNally, 1964. Pp. 224—229.
6. Olson, M., Jr.   *The Logic of Collective Action.* Cambridge: Harvard University Press, 1965. Pp. 5—8.
7. Nursing Development Conference Group.   Minutes of the first meeting (typewritten), Sept. 6, 1968. P. 1.
8. de Montcheuil, Y.   *Guide for Social Action.* Chicago: Fides Publishers, 1954. Pp. 21—23.
9. King, A. R., Jr., and Brownell, J. A.   *The Curriculum and the Disciplines of Knowledge.* New York: Wiley, 1966. Pp. 68—71.

2

Frames of Reference in Nursing

The members of the NDCG adhere to the position that nursing's enduring contributions to society are in part dependent upon the formalization and validation of theoretical and practical knowledge to guide nurses' actions. The experiences of the authors support the importance of nurses' development and use of conceptual frameworks in all areas of nursing endeavor.

Nursing's logically structured body of knowledge should be a source of the components of various frames of reference used by nurses in nursing practice, education, research and development, theorizing, and scholarly endeavors. At the same time nurses' engagement in these endeavors should contribute to the formulation, expression, and structuring of views, concepts, values, and modes of action to guide or regulate what nurses do in society. Giving form and structure to nursing's domain of knowledge would make an enduring contribution to all areas of nursing endeavor because nursing knowledge is the element common to all the areas of endeavor necessary to maintain nursing in a society (see Fig. 1-1).

The emphasis in the 1970s on nurses' use of conceptual frameworks to guide nursing practice and education seems to (1) suggest that nursing knowledge is already well defined and logically structured and (2) assume that nurses have formulated and expressed their insights about and conceptualizations of nursing in the form of stable and appropriate structures that can be communicated using existing symbol systems or language. Since both nursing and nursing education are in formative stages of development as disciplines of knowledge, their domains and boundaries and conceptual systems are not well defined and the symbol system for expressing nursing concepts is relatively undeveloped.

The emphasis in the 1970s on the use of conceptual frameworks to guide nursing practice, nursing education, and nursing research is viewed as a continuation of earlier movements in nursing and in education. One example is the nationwide movement for the integration of mental health concepts into nursing curricula. Another example is the post-Sputnik movement in the U.S.A. to improve the teaching of the sciences and mathematics. This movement led specialists in a number of sciences to look at the structure of their respective disciplines to identify the key ideas and conceptual constructs that students should attend to in the process of mastering knowledge in the science.

It is the advanced scholars in any field whose psychologically structured knowledge conforms to the state of development and structuring of the knowledge specific to that field. Nursing scholars, therefore, have a primary responsibility to contribute to the laying out of the domain and boundaries of nursing knowledge, to specify the forms of nursing knowledge, and to develop its conceptual structure. This is no small task. It involves the laying out of the views, concepts, and values that are significant for nurses who function in that *sector of reality* that constitutes the "world of the nurse" (i.e., the areas of human affairs and the human phenomena with respect to which nurses operate as nurses and for which they bear responsibility in a society). Scholars, researchers, and theorists then must identify, describe, and explain *what the nurse is concerned with* within this sector of reality and *in what way the nurse is concerned.* This is the *sector of nursing science* [1]. Without frames of reference that have their foundations in organized nursing knowledge, nurses do not have adequate bases for (1) isolating significant phenomena, (2) evaluating data, (3) communicating ideas, and (4) regulating their actions in society [2].

The purpose of this chapter is to offer some ideas for clarification and resolution of problems and issues regarding the characteristics and the process of development of frames of reference to guide nursing practice and nursing education. In the process, a focus will be maintained on the domain and dimensions of nursing as a discipline of knowledge (a practice discipline) and as practical endeavor.

PRELIMINARY CONSIDERATIONS

Since the 1950s nurses have been involved in a concerted way with exploration of various dimensions of nursing with emphasis on its social, interpersonal, and health aspects [3—21]. This has included the formulation, expression, and naming of concepts that point to or explain the realities of nursing practice. The mandate of the 1970s that nursing curricula be developed from explicit conceptual frameworks suggests a culmination of the earlier (and continuing) efforts of nurses to weave social, interpersonal, and health concepts and values into the fabric of nursing and nursing education [22]. This continued focus on structures of concepts and values suggests that nursing may be approaching the point of coming of age as a practice discipline and as a profession.

The work of structuring conceptual frameworks for purposes of nursing education and nursing practice has taken different forms, and the products known to the writers vary in both composition and complexity. Sometimes the result is a listing(s) of concepts without order or structure, or the naming of three or four concepts with no identification of relationships among them. Or the product may be a hierarchical structure of concepts arranged in an order from the most general to the specific and factual; sometimes it is a network type of structure of related concepts or sets of such structures. The time-honored concepts of man, society, and health have a place in many of the frameworks [20, pp. 22—23]. And sometimes it seems that the process rather than the product becomes the primary focus of the framework developer.

Engagement in the processes of development of conceptual or other frames of reference is costly in terms of both time and energy of individuals. It is, however, a most intellectually rewarding endeavor that can bring great practical returns to both nurses and society. Nurses who have found that specific concepts, structures of related concepts, or expressions of views and values have utility in nursing practice and education will no doubt continue in the endeavors of structuring frames of reference. But will the results of the expenditures of time, energy, and money to isolate concepts and build conceptual frameworks be put to use more generally toward the continued development of nursing and nursing education as practice disciplines? Will the flurry of activity in the 1970s to formulate and express the concepts that form the underlying and supportive structure of nursing die down, or will activity be intensified toward the clarification of nursing's domain, its boundaries, and the structuring of its various areas of knowledge — both theoretical and practical? If the activity dies down quickly as does a rain shower, the advancement of nursing toward its potential as a service in society will continue to be delayed and the substantive materials essential for nursing education will continue to be ill defined. What occurs rests with nurses, for only nurses can move their own discipline.

The NDCG's attempt to clarify some of the problems and issues regarding frames of reference for nursing emphasizes products as well as process. Thinking in this regard has been guided by the admonition — to go is to *move from,* to get there is *to have.* Where to begin, how to proceed, and what is "created" are questions specific to the endeavors of framework development. These are the questions that served to give focus to subsequent expressions of ideas about development of frames of reference for nursing purposes.

Sections of the chapter address (1) the process of framework development in nursing, (2) conditions that affect nurses' engagement in framework development or their use of developed and expressed frames of reference, and (3) some issues and problems related to nursing frames of reference.

FRAMEWORK DEVELOPMENT
An Overview
As indicated, a central problem in the development of frames of reference for nursing is where, how, and with what does a developer begin. Orem in 1973 [23] suggested that con-

ceptual framework development in nursing can begin by nurses attending to the most general conceptualizations of man and society that can subsume nursing. A design for a general frame of reference to guide nursing scholars who seek to uncover nursing's conceptual frames of reference is presented in Figure 2-1.

Orem's broad subsuming general framework for nursing is constituted from three interlocking frames. The frames are named in order from the most general to the least general:

1. Nursing's Placement in the World of Man
2. Nursing's Placement in Human Affairs
3. Nursing

Two elements of the framework serve central articulating functions in linking the three frames. "Fields of Knowledge and Human Endeavor" articulates Frame 1 with Frame 2; and "Nursing" articulates Frame 2 with Frame 3. For the understanding scholar, the three frames represent conceptual clusters for use in organizing available knowledge in a way that is meaningful for nursing purposes.

For example, in one university school of nursing curriculum, units were designed and developed as a mechanism to guide the nursing faculty in the structuring of nursing and nursing-related knowledge. The names of six curriculum design units reflect some of the insights about nursing expressed or implicit in Figure 2-1. The curriculum design units were identified as: (1) Nursing, a Practice Discipline; (2) the Professional Nurse Practitioner and Scholar; (3) Nursing, a Health Service; (4) Nursing, an Assisting (helping) Service; (5) Nursing: Demand for and Technologies and Forms of by Categories of Cases; (6) Nursing Practice Related to Individuals, a Number of Individuals During the Same Time Period, Small Groups [24].

In Orem's suggested general frame of reference for nursing, Frame 1, "Nursing's Placement in the World of Man," identifies that the generic term *man* (and the developer's concept of man) subsumes both (individual) "Human Beings" and "Human Groups." The frame identifies two triads or con-

22

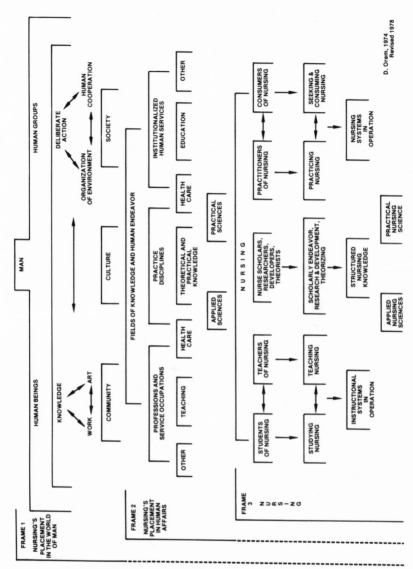

Figure 2-1 Nursing's placement in the world of man and human affairs.

structs that characterize individuals and groups with respect to (1) generation of the sociologically named elements (i.e., Community, Culture, Society), and (2) development of or engagement in specific "Fields of Knowledge and Human Endeavor." These two triads "Knowledge — Work — Art" and "Deliberate Action — Organization of Environment — Human Cooperation" express the human foundations for all framework elements identified in Frame 2, nursing included.

Frame 2 should be seen as a construct developed because of its relevance to *Nursing,* not as an exhaustive development of "Fields of Knowledge and Human Endeavor." The structural and functional entities named in Frame 2, namely, "Professions and Service Occupations," "Practice Disciplines," and "Institutionalized Human Services" are expressed at a level of generality such that descriptive or explanatory knowledge about each would be relevant to all professions, service occupations, practice disciplines, and human services. Frame 2 further identifies and narrows nursing's placement in human affairs by specifying that nursing fits into the professions through "teaching" and "health care" and into human services through "education" and "health care." In both instances there is indication of the recognition of the existence of professions and services that are not nursing through the use of "other." In Frame 2, "Practice Disciplines" are recognized as being constituted of two kinds of knowledge, "theoretical" and "practical," which when logically structured would constitute the applied and the practical nursing sciences.

In the general frame of reference for nursing formulated and used by Orem the elements named in Frame 3, "Nursing," are subsumed by the conceptualizations expressed in both Frames 1 and 2. Frame 3 is developed in three sections. The central section is organized around *nursing knowledge* and the two side sections around *nursing education* and *nursing practice.* In working within Frame 3 it should be understood that *nursing education* and *nursing practice* can be viewed from both the perspectives of "Professions" and of "Human Services"; and nurse scholars, researchers, and others can be viewed from the perspective of "Profession" or "Practice Discipline."

Figure 2-1 is offered as an outcome of the first stage of development of conceptual frameworks for nursing. The concern of this stage (from Orem's perspective) is the reality placement of nursing and general limit setting for nursing. Frames 1 and 2 in the figure are viewed as providing answers to the question: How does nursing fit into the world of man and human affairs? The framework developer who asks the question, *"Do these frames of reference subsume the nursing elements in Frame 3?"* should be able to answer *Yes* or *No*.

Conceptual framework development for nursing purposes is assumed to be a learning process. The developer as learner works with data, develops insights, and formulates and verifies hypotheses. Learning is an unfolding and a growth of concepts analogous to development of living things [25].

Where to Begin, How to Proceed

Conceptual frameworks are cognitive structures, products that result from the observations, inferences, insights, and conceptualizations of experienced and creative individuals in a field of endeavor. To be shared with other individuals, a conceptual framework must be expressed in propositions or in word models. Expression of the conceptual parts and relationships among the parts of a framework requires an adequate symbol system or language. An individual's state of readiness to work with abstractions including relationships will determine in part what that person can do in formulating and structuring frames of reference. The absence of language adequate for expressing the conceptualized parts of a framework will present problems to the framework formulator, and the introduction of new terms (naming theory) to symbolize the real world referents of conceptualized parts of a framework may present problems to individuals who engage in the scholarly endeavor of studying an expressed framework. But the central problem remains: Where, how, and with what does framework formation begin?

If Orem's expressed general frame of reference for nursing is accepted, framework developers would direct attention to endeavors that result in an unfolding and growth of cognitive structures to characterize and explain nursing in its specificity (Frame 3) and in terms of characteristics that describe nursing as well as other fields of endeavor (Frames 1 and 2). Conceptual frameworks for nursing are viewed not as the totality of formulated, expressed, and structured nursing knowledge but as being constituted from concepts that function together to give direction and form to the discovery, structuring, and use of nursing knowledge. Concepts that function in this fashion have the power to organize other concepts and to move the thinking of a nurse to a more complex point of view based upon new integrations of knowledge and the emergence of new structures. For example, Figure 2-1 viewed as a frame of reference is relatively undifferentiated; movement in framework development would be recognized through the production of more differentiated and more specific frames of reference.

Where to Begin   A developer can begin to work in any one of the three frames of Figure 2-1 or can do concurrent work in each one. To facilitate understanding of nursing's general characteristics, it is suggested that Frame 2 of Figure 2-1, "Nursing's Placement in Human Affairs," is a desirable starting point. While general, the entities within the frame, upon investigation, can lead to the development of insights, views, concepts, and values that are as specific to nursing as they are to other "professions and service occupations," "practice disciplines," and "human services." Definitive endeavors in framework development could begin with scholarly investigation of the authoritative literature specific to the most general entities named in Frame 2. Such investigation can begin with *professions* or *practice disciplines* or *human services* but eventually must be extended to all three with attention being given to the relationships among them.

For example, a framework developer who takes the position that nursing has had,[1] has, or is moving toward the status of a *profession* and who explores and analyzes the literature

---

[1] See Stinson, S. M. *Deprofessionalization in nursing.* Columbia University, Teachers College Ed. D., 1959 (unpublished).

> *Proposition 1.* Each profession exists in a society so that its members can identify, diagnose, resolve, and solve or mitigate a specific class of human problems of members of the society.
>
> *Proposition 2.* The class of human problems specific to each profession constitutes the profession's domain of practice in the society.
>
> *Proposition 3.* The class of human problems that serves to specify a profession's domain of practice points to the human and social and environmental phenomena about which the members of the profession must acquire and accumulate knowledge.
>
> *Proposition 4.* The class of human problems that serves to specify a profession's domain of practice also specifies the areas of theoretical and practical knowledge that must be developed, structured, and mastered by members of the profession.
>
> *Proposition 5.* Each profession to perpetuate itself and to progress in serving a society must have members engaged (a) in rendering service to individuals and groups in the society who can be helped through it, (b) in the education of new members, (c) in research and in development of techniques and technologies of practice, and (d) in theory formulation to advance knowledge about the dimensions of human problems that occasion the profession's existence.

Figure 2-2 Characteristics of professions.

on the professions and engages in reflection may arrive at significant insights and conclusions and be in a position to formulate and express basic ideas and propositions about the professions. An example of a result of such a process is presented in Figure 2-2 in the form of a set of propositions about the characteristics of *professions.* The key ideas expressed in the five propositions are (1) classes of human problems, (2) domains of practice, (3) theoretical and practical knowledge, (4) essential functions of members of a profession, and (5) the distribution of functions to members of a profession.

Another suggested movement is an analysis of the expressed ideas or the stated propositions about the entity under study.

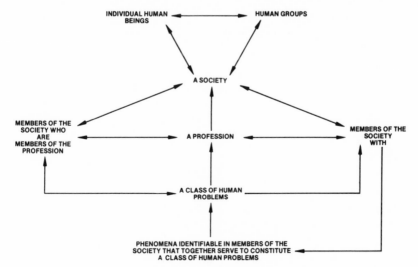

Figure 2-3   The professions are human problems focused.

Figure 2-3 is the result of an analysis of the first proposition in Figure 2-2 to lay out the key ideas within the proposition and the relationships among them. Figure 2-3 also indicates articulation with entities from Frame 1, namely, "Society," "Individual Human Beings," and "Human Groups."

In analyzing the key ideas or stated propositions about professions or practice disciplines or institutionalized human services, it is helpful to identify elements common to all the expressed ideas or propositions. For example, in the five propositions about the professions the element that is named in each proposition is "class of human problems." It is the class of human problems specific to a profession that defines both its domain of knowledge and service.

While working within the context of Frame 2, the investigator also can ask the question: "What view(s) of man is implicit in the frame?" If scholarly investigation has attained a sufficient degree of specificity, the developer may have arrived at a level of understanding that provides the answer (i.e., *man in need of help* and *man as helper* [14, pp. 69–73]). These correlative views of man add specificity to the element's professions, practice disciplines, and human services.

The two views of man, *man as helper* and *man in need of help,* are related views. The relationship between them can be described and explained in terms of the differences in the conditions of persons characterized as in need of help and as helpers and the complementary nature of these conditions. *Helping relationships* and *helping processes* are the man-made forces that bind such persons together as functioning unities. Conceptualization of persons and relationships from this perspective provides a frame of reference helpful to nurses and others.

The formulation and expression of the "helping construct" (Fig. 2-4) organized around the two expressed views of man is a movement toward framework complexity and specificity. The construct articulates Frame 2 elements under investigation with Frame 1 elements. Furthermore, the helping construct provides a frame of reference for theory development, research, and further scholarly investigation leading to the identification, validation, and organization of a body of knowledge about helping — a body of knowledge important to all the helping professions and human services.

How to Proceed, Frames 1 and 2 It is suggested that there is no fixed pathway for movement toward more specific framework development with respect to *nursing's placement*

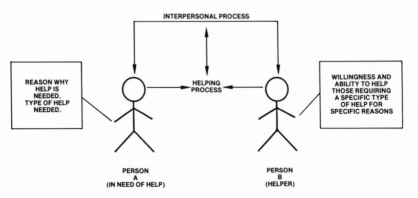

Figure 2-4 The helping construct.

in the world of man and human affairs (Frames 1 and 2) Fig. 2—1). The suggestions offered about where to begin may have some value in setting directions. However, it is the interests, concerns, and the relevant scholarly achievements of framework developers that will give direction to their initial expenditures of energy and their modes of advancement.

A number of suggestions about procedure related to cognitive movement in Frames 1 and 2 are offered on the basis of experience, with a minimum of justification and discussion.

1. Explication of the view of *man as agent* as the most general view of man implicit in Frame 2
2. Understanding that a concept of *man as agent* subsumes concepts of *man as helper* and *man in need of help*
3. Understanding the named views of man within the frames of reference provided by the constructs
   a. Knowledge — Work — Art
   b. Deliberate Action — Organization of Environment — Human Cooperation
   c. Community — Culture — Society
4. Understanding ways of categorizing Fields of Knowledge and Human Endeavor within the frame of reference of western civilization or within other frames of reference
5. Inquiry into Fields of Knowledge and Human Endeavor within the frames of reference provided by Professions and Service Occupations — Practice Disciplines — Institutionalized Human Services
6. Inquiry into Health Care and Education within the frame of reference of Human Services; and into Health Care and Teaching within the frame of reference of Professions and Service Occupations
7. Inquiry into nursing's fit within Health Care and Education (service frame of reference) and within Health Care and Teaching (profession frame of reference)
8. Inquiry into Practice Discipline with respect to Theoretical and Practical knowledge components
9. Understanding nursing as a practice discipline, a body of knowledge with theoretical and practical knowledge components both of which have utility to guide the investigatory and regulatory actions of nurses in nursing practice
10. Inquiry into the ways in which nurses have described nursing's sector of reality (world of the nurse) and nursing's sector of science (what the world of the nurse is concerned with and in what way it is concerned)

How to Proceed, Frame 3 Movement from frames of reference descriptive and explanatory of nursing's placement in the world of man and human affairs to the development of frames of reference specific to nursing (as contrasted with nursing's shared frames of reference) demands willingness on the part of framework developers to accept nursing as a specific and unique entity in a society. This means that a framework developer who is able to think about nursing as a profession or a practice discipline or a human service or a health service or as all these must now become able to inquire into what nurses are concerned with as nurses and how they are concerned. Nursing's focus or proper object in the world of the nurse must be explicated. A nursing rationale must be expressed in answer to the question: "What human conditions generate requirements for nursing?"

Movement toward the development of the conceptual frameworks and views of man specific to nursing is an initial movement in the psychologic structuring of a body or bodies of nursing knowledge. Nursing considered as a field of knowledge is poorly organized. As previously mentioned, this affects courses of action that nurses will decide to take. Nurses who are advanced scholars in fields such as physiology, anthropology, or sociology may not have advanced as nursing scholars, having remained in some instances at the level of scholarship in nursing attained in an initial nursing program. The effective conceptual framework developer in nursing is first and foremost a nursing scholar who has conceptualized the view(s) of man that are nursing specific.

Movement within Frame 3 may be facilitated by exploration and analysis of nurses' expressed definitions and generalizations about nursing (see Chap. 4). Movement, however, cannot be definitive without the acceptance of a general theory or concept of nursing that identifies the reality focus of nursing and the broad conceptual structure of nursing. Such a conceptual structure would subsume not only facts about nursing as it has been and is practiced but also would express that which nursing can and should become in a society. The reader is referred to Chapter 6 for a description

of the kinds of endeavors engaged in and the conceptual structures that resulted from the NDCG's use of one general theory
of nursing.

Summary
Conceptual framework development has been identified as a
cognitive developmental type of process. The process has
been described as an unfolding, a movement of growth in
insight and conceptualization in which new integrations occur.
Ideas and arrangements among ideas become more intri-
cate.

The use of a general frame of reference for understanding
nursing in relation to its placement in the world of man and
human affairs (Fig. 2-1) is suggested. The essential idea be-
hind the offering of Figure 2-1 is that it is important to see
and come to understand the broad dimensions of a frame of
reference for nursing before expending effort to develop segments of it. From a developmental or learning perspective,
this is analogous to movement from the *simple to the complex* (i.e., movement from the relatively undifferentiated to
the more detailed, more specific, more interrelated, and
therefore more complex).

Where to begin and how to proceed in the development of
frames of reference for nursing are viewed as problem areas
for framework developers. Of critical concern from the perspective of organized nursing is the availability of advanced
nursing scholars who are able and willing to expend the necessary time, and to make the effort that is primarily intellectual.

USING CONCEPTUAL FRAMES OF REFERENCE
Framework Orientations
Frames of reference used by nurses may be primarily oriented
toward work, person, need, health, disease, adaptation, or
system. The orientations of nurses' frames of reference can
be understood in relation to their foundational and continuing education in nursing and in nursing-related fields; their
nursing experiences; their relationships with nurse colleagues

and with colleagues in other fields; their education in the liberal arts and humanities; their interests and concerns as these relate to espoused views of man, the world, and the universe; and, of course, the range of their life experiences. Of critical importance to nursing students are the cues offered to them by nurse teachers who move them to discover and organize the views, concepts, and systems of values that prove helpful in guiding their actions as nurses.

The use by nurses of conceptual frames of reference specific to nursing is not so frequently encountered as is their use of the outright medical frame of reference with its focus on man as *subject to disease and injury.* This condition in nursing is due in part to the relatively unorganized state of nursing as a discipline of knowledge (a field of inquiry) and to the variations in nurses' understandings of nursing's proper object or focus in a society. Teachers of nursing have a major role in helping students to develop the ability to *think nursing,* not just to interact with patients and provide measures of care according to specified rules and procedures which at times are without explicit rationales.

The use of theories of nursing that lay out the views, concepts, and systems of values that are *nursing specific* is essential for both effective nursing practice and nursing education. Frames of reference that are common to the health-care and other helping professions and services are of value to nurses but are not adequate for nursing purposes. Some nurses practice nursing with a nursing frame of reference that is implicit in their thinking and their care activities but never have made their frames of reference explicit. As one expert nurse clinician said, "I would like to know" the theory that underlies my practice. The communication of one's nursing views, concepts, and values to others is not possible without such knowledge. It is the questioning intelligence of individual nurses that exerts the greatest influence on the use and continuing development of conceptual frames of reference. The subsequent account by one NDCG member of her personal experiences is of interest in this regard.[2]

[2] Judy Crews.

This account, as well as accounts from other nurses, points out that when a nurse *functions without an explicit and valid theory of nursing* the nurse tends to seek out forms of action that the nursing community holds out as high-level practice. The forms of action and roles elected by the nurse (e.g. patient advocate, coordinator of care) are, in a sense, rationalizations of the nurse's dissatisfactions with her or his intellectual growth as nursing practitioner.

A PERSONAL EXPERIENCE

On a baccalaureate level in the late 1950s I learned to focus on the "Seven Basic Needs" of man or the "Comprehensive Approach" to nursing care. I found this approach helpful in identifying areas of knowledge and patient problems with which to be concerned. However, there were some frustrations. The approaches were both vague and rigid. They were vague in that the areas of "need" as outlined didn't seem to lead to specific frameworks of nursing action. They were rigid in that I was given the expectation that I had to identify, for example, the "emotional needs" of patients. But suppose I couldn't observe any emotional needs? If a patient disclaimed any emotional problems and I couldn't describe any, was it true he or she didn't have any difficulties in this area — or were my lack of experience and naiveté leading to an erroneous conclusion? How could I analyze a patient's health-care problem to predict or project the emotional effects? How could I justify probing the personality and internal life of a patient without a nursing framework to guide in the formulation of appropriate nursing outcome goals? I didn't have the answers to these questions and since nobody was pressing me to discover them I put them aside.

My first few years as a nurse saw me focusing in on and gaining specific clinical nursing skills and gaining a confident self-image as a provider of nursing care. I saw nursing then in the early sixties as patient-centered. I saw the nurse as a caring professional using clusters of knowledge to guide in the provision of care and using certain needed techniques doing this within an emotionally supportive relationship between patient and nurse. I also saw the nurse as the patient advocate in that the nurse was protective, was a communicator, coordinator, and priority setter functioning between the patient and the environment including all those who interacted with the patient.

After these early professional goals were met there developed a personal need to get more involved with in-depth nursing practice, remaining with patients. A temporary solution, as it was, and still is, for many other nurses, was to practice intensive-care nursing and master increasingly complex medical and nursing technologies. But acute-care nursing eventually led to more frustration. There was no movement and no creativity associated with my work as I continued the practice of intensive-care nursing. I asked: "Is the maximum contribution that I can make to patients and nursing the expenditure of my best possible efforts over an 8-hour work day? *Can I continue doing this without making a contribution to the further development of nursing in the interests of these and other patients?"*

During this period I experienced the desire for graduate education in nursing and sought and achieved a master's degree. Finally, I moved to being in a state of readiness to be willing to work with a theoretical framework for nursing.

Conditions Affecting Use of a Conceptual Framework

After a number of experiences with groups of clinical nurse specialists, one NDCG member expressed some of her observations and inferences as follows:

1. The desire for a conceptual framework for nursing comes from a practitioner's experiencing the need for guides to aid the search for and the organization of patient information significant for nursing purposes.
2. A nurse's use of a general theory of nursing provides a basis for and enhances the autonomy of the nurse.[3]
3. A general theory of nursing with its specific conceptual structure will be used in different ways by practitioners of nursing and to different extents and depths.

Another NDCG member, on the basis of her experiences with individual nurses and groups of nurses in educational and practice settings, summarized characteristics of persons with interests in developing or working with a framework of nursing concepts. Such persons were identified as:

1. *Dissatisfied* with the status quo (i.e., with the lack of a coherent conceptual structure), experiencing a felt need for a conceptual framework in nursing as a basis for education, practice, and research
2. *Willing* to listen with an open mind to proposed ideas or to discussions of theories of nursing with specific conceptual structures
3. *Able to tolerate* the initial confusion and stress associated with actively incorporating a new conceptual structure within one's psychologically structured knowledge and to reorganize one's accumulated theoretical and practical nursing knowledge around it

[3] In a different situation a graduate student in nursing expressed an observation made about herself in these words, "Don't you know it sets me free?"

4. *In need* of a great deal of guidance and support in trying to work with a conceptual framework and to use it in nursing practice or teaching or research. Support may be in the form of consultations, publications, and so forth. Highly conceptual, independent thinkers may work alone (but group support is important here) or in groups in further development of conceptual frameworks.

It was also demonstrated that some nurses may experience ambivalence about using conceptual frameworks to guide their nursing and teaching actions. Interest may lag in expending effort to use or further develop a framework when demands of daily living leave little time or energy available for such purposes.

The NDCG members have also identified factors and conditions that block or interfere with nurses' development and use of conceptual frames of reference specific to nursing.

1. Questions of friends or colleagues in the field about the relevance or importance of conceptual frames of reference that are nursing specific
2. What others think and express about a specific general theory of nursing and the conceptual frames of reference it provides
3. Belief that one must have "permission" to use a specific conceptual frame of reference in nursing
4. Prevailing modes of thought about nursing operating on the premise that nursing as an outcome or a product is well defined and understood by all nurses and the only task to be done is to outline the activities that nurses should perform
5. Absence of an experiencing of need — "There is no need. I am getting along O.K." or "I know this as a nurse; there is no need to make this explicit, to share it with others."
6. Conditions in work situations that do not promote the use or development of explicit nursing frames of reference
7. Fear on part of nurses of becoming involved or committing themselves to the use of a specific nursing theory
8. Wanting to use a nursing theory but not wanting to expend time and effort in understanding its conceptual structure; or to be involved in its application
9. Rejection of terms that are used to express the conceptual elements of a nursing theory without inquiry into their meaning within the theory or the reasons for their use
10. Misuse of terms because of lack of insight about their referents

11. Not being realistic about the knowledge and the skills or the effort and time necessary for the development and use of frames of reference specific to nursing

Reflection upon the foregoing expressions of conditions and factors that facilitate or block nurses' development or use of conceptual and other frames of reference specific to nursing may lead to a number of conclusions. This exercise is left to the reader.

PROBLEMS AND ISSUES
Some problems and issues in nursing that are associated with the development, use, and continued development of views, concepts, and values that constitute nurses' frames of reference are expressed. Five problems and three issues identified and expressed by NDCG members have been selected for presentation to and consideration by the nursing community.

Problems
The problems are expressed in terms of situations that are seen as resulting in uncertainty on the part of nurses about ways to reach decisions on courses of action to be taken in the development and use of nursing frames of reference, especially conceptual frames of reference. The problems are expressed as follows:

1. The situation of organized nursing in which there is a lack of clear-cut guidelines for the development and use of conceptual frames of reference that are specific to nursing
2. The situation of having available to nurses nursing knowledge with a range of degrees of validity but having this knowledge in a relatively unorganized state and widely scattered in the periodical literature
3. The situation of need in the nursing community for the development and use of strategies to help nurses understand and accept nursing as a discipline of knowledge and not just a field of practice
4. The situation of failure within organized nursing and within university schools of nursing to afford high priority to and to value and reward endeavors associated with the formulation of the logical structure of nursing knowledge

5. Situations in nursing education where faculties or instructional staffs formulate, express, and structure ideas to serve to identify and articulate components of a curriculum but (for a range of reasons) do not adequately use these ideas in development of curriculum designs or in the selection and articulation of instructional experiences for nursing students

These problems are viewed as in need of both resolution and solution. If they are unattended to by the nursing community they will increase in complexity and become more serious as sources of difficulty in decision-making. Some suggestions for ways and means used by the NDCG and its members to resolve and solve these problems are presented in subsequent chapters.

Issues

It has been noted by NDCG members as well as by others that the promulgation of different positions about nursing frames of reference or their sources by members of the nursing community affects decisions being made about the frames of reference used by nurses to guide their nursing endeavors. Three cases of opposing points of view are presented.

Issue 1.   *Nurses do* (the NDCG's position), *nurses do not* require a cognitional orientation to nursing in the form of theories, conceptual constructs, laws, and rules that elaborate nursing's focus in a society or describe and explain the realities with which nurses deal and set forth how and why they are concerned with these realities.

Issue 2.   *Nursing theories are general theories of man variously expressed* versus *nursing theories are grounded in the general characteristics of nursing and in the realities that nurses deal with as nurses; the view(s) of man specific to nursing is discernible in these realities and in the relationships among them* (the NDCG's position).

Issue 3.   *Nursing is not a science and can never be developed as a science* versus *nursing is a pure science* versus *nursing*

knowledge can be developed as a set of applied sciences and a practical science (the NDCG's position).

The three issues selected for presentation are ones that are significant with respect to nurses' endeavors directed toward the goal of structuring nursing knowledge. Their significance rests in the kinds of decisions that nurses who adhere to these various positions have made and will make with respect to the future development of nursing. Some approaches to the resolution of the issues are presented in subsequent chapters.

REFERENCES

1. O'Doherty, E. F. Minutes of the May 20, 1965, Meeting of the Nursing Model Committee and the Faculty of Nursing, The Catholic University of America, Washington, D.C. P. 1 (typewritten).
2. *The Random House Dictionary of the English Language* (unabridged) New York: Random House, 1973. P. 563.
3. Peplau, H. E. *Interpersonal Relations in Nursing: A Conceptual Frame of Reference for Psychodynamic Nursing.* New York: G. P. Putnam's, 1952.
4. Orem, D. E. *Guides for Developing Curricula for the Education of Practical Nurses.* Washington, D.C.: U.S. Government Printing Office, 1959.
5. Gifford, A. (Ed.). *Unity of Nursing Care.* Chapel Hill: The University of North Carolina School of Nursing, 1960.
6. Abdellah, F. G., Beland, I., Martin, A., and Matheney, R. *Patient-Centered Approaches to Nursing.* New York: Macmillan, 1960.
7. Orlando, I. J. *The Dynamic Nurse-Patient Relationship.* New York: Putnam's, 1961.
8. Johnson, D. E. The significance of nursing care. *Am. J. Nurs.* 61: 63–66, 1961.
9. Wiedenbach, E. *Clinical Nursing: A Helping Art.* New York: Springer Publishing Co., 1964.
10. Wald, F. S., and Leonard, R. C. Towards development of nursing practice theory. *Nurs. Res.* 13:309–313, 1964.
11. Henderson, V. *The Nature of Nursing.* New York: Macmillan, 1966.
12. King, I. M. A conceptual frame of reference for nursing. *Nurs. Res.* 17:27–31, 1968.
13. Rogers, M. *An Introduction to the Theoretical Basis of Nursing.* Philadelphia: Davis, 1970.
14. Orem, D. E. *Nursing: Concepts of Practice.* New York: McGraw-Hill, 1971.

15. Stevens, B. J.   Analysis of structural forms used in nursing curricula. *Nurs. Res.* 20:388–397, 1971.

16. Longway, I. M.   Curriculum Concepts — An Historical Analysis. *Nurs. Outlook* 20:116–117, 1972.

17. Hodgman, E. A.   Conceptual framework to guide nursing curriculum. *Nurs. Forum* 12:110–131, 1973.

18. Nursing Development Conference Group.   *Concept Formalization in Nursing: Process and Product.* Boston: Little, Brown, 1973.

19. Riehl, J. P., and Roy, C.   *Conceptual Models for Nursing Practice.* New York: Appleton-Century-Crofts, 1974.

20. National League for Nursing, Department of Baccalaureate and Higher Degree Programs. Faculty-Curriculum Development.   Part III. *Conceptual Framework — Its Meaning and Function* (Pub. No. 15-1558). New York: National League for Nursing, 1975.

21. Chater, S. C.   A conceptual framework for curriculum development. *Nurs. Outlook* 23:428–433, 1975.

22. National League for Nursing, Department of Baccalaureate and Higher Degree Programs.   *Criteria for the Appraisal of Baccalaureate and Higher Degree Programs in Nursing* (Pub. No. 15-1215). New York: National League for Nursing, 1972. P. 8.

23. Orem, D. E.   Process in the development of a conceptual framework for teaching and for the practice of nursing. Presented at the Institute on Conceptual Frameworks, Washington, D.C., The School of Nursing, The Catholic University of America, Oct. 5, 1973.

24. Orem, D. E.   Curriculum Design. Memorandum to the Curriculum Project Staff of the Georgetown University School of Nursing (typewritten), Washington, D.C., May 11, 1971.

25. Lonergan, B. J. F.   *Insight.* New York: Philosophical Library, 1958. Pp. 286, 461, 470–471.

3

Nursing: A Practice Discipline

The initial concern of the NDCG has been the process of formalization and structuring of nursing knowledge. Our efforts have been based on the assumption that nursing is a potential discipline of knowledge awaiting the continued, concerted, and disciplined efforts of nurses to identify and describe the domain of nursing, the boundaries thereof, and to formulate or structure its fundamental ideas.

Disciplines are dynamic species of knowledge, structures of inquiry and understanding emerging from continual processes of development. The disciplines manifest the *discovered* patterns of possible development in knowledge. In every discipline many such patterns can be presumed to await discovery [1]. Nursing, as a discipline of knowledge, is beginning to manifest articulated theories or patterns that are guiding inquiry and the development of new nursing knowledge as well as providing a logical framework for connecting what is done in practice with theory, which helps to describe, explain, and predict.

The purpose of this chapter is to present ideas that will aid nurses in their construction of frames of reference for approaching nursing as a practice discipline. Components of such frames of reference are derived from (1) understanding of the function of concepts in discipline development (including general concepts); (2) the frame of reference of science, including the structure of nursing sciences; and (3) theory in nursing. Key ideas from these three areas are presented.

CONCEPTS AND DISCIPLINE DEVELOPMENT

Inquiry, or directed thinking, has its origin in a conceptual structure. In a science a conception, borrowed or invented by the inquirer(s), serves as a guide to the collection of relevant and important data [2]. Nursing phenomena tend to confound us by the great variety of characteristics, qualities, behaviors, and interactions that they present to our view. Therefore, it is essential that adequate conceptions, which may form the substantive structure of nursing as a scientific discipline and which may guide inquiry, be discovered, invented, and articulated adequately.

Concept Formalization in Disciplines

A concept is the product of persons observing instances (e.g., of nursing) with their regularities and variants, thinking about these real-world phenomena, and finding in them unexpected likenesses of structure, unity, and intelligibility [3]. Concepts may be described as extensions of percepts, as a grasp of overall structure obtained by the isolation and identification of relevant factors and relationships in orderly array [4, 5]. Conceptualizing about nursing, then, *enables us to cast the complex phenomena observed in nursing cases and situations into manageable models or simplified approximations of the real world of nursing.*

A concept may be communicated verbally by giving a definition of the symbol, which is its name. A definition of nursing consists of an explicit statement that conveys the meaning or the connotation of the term *nursing.* To be clear, such a definition should enumerate the minimum number of qualities in its connotation sufficient to identify the term unambiguously [6].

The units in which the messages are written — the concepts that form the substantive structure of nursing — must be found, discovered, searched out. They are not immediately self-evident. (The NDCG's concept of nursing system presented in this book is the result of such deliberative endeavor.)

Deliberate effort is required to set forth a general concept of what nursing is. Such a concept is the product of persons observing instances of nursing, thinking about these events, and finding likenesses among them, discovering that which gives these events unity and intelligibility. Individuals search for distinct elements or units that are invariants in the society or in the persons nursed, for likenesses of structure, and for how the elements are related or organized into the whole.

A well-defined concept of nursing will be an accurate *tool for thinking and dealing with the real world of nursing* only if it is referrable to actual stimulus situations. A concept, embodied in a definition, *permits generalizations to be made by which one may respond to a group of instances, or a class as a whole in terms of some abstract property,* and may also *discriminate between classes of stimuli* even in novel stimulus situations [7]. Adequate definitions or expressed general concepts of nursing will (1) hold for all instances of nursing and (2) be translatable into propositions with the form, "if X (a requirement for nursing) exists then Y is observable," Y being the factors and the relationships among them that generate the known condition that can be regulated through nursing. Nursing is a unique service in society. American society provides for the specialized roles of a number of health workers including those of nurses, as well as for institutionalized ways to provide nursing and prepare practitioners. The nurse performs socially prescribed functions in the area of health-care services. Although the nurse's tasks are linked to, and may be the same as, those performed by others in health-care services, the uniqueness of nursing lies in the *reasons for* what the nurse does in society as well as in the characteristics of what is done. A description of the why and what of nursing would embody a general concept of nursing and would constitute a guide for inquiry and for the structuring of nursing knowledge.

In a practice discipline[1] such as nursing, a general concept is necessary to guide behavior of nurses in the *production of results.* Conceptualizations regarding the essential structure of nursing are needed by the *scholar,* the *researcher,* the *practitioner,* and the *student of nursing* so that each can respond to various types of nursing experience in relatively stable ways without being faced with the chaos of treating each new experience with a totally new response [7, p. 50; 8]. A general concept of nursing is a necessary tool to *organize nursing reality* and to be able to look at this reality

[1] A practice discipline is practical science, a body of knowledge concerned with bringing about practical results — some range of purposeful changes in or control of real-life situations.

differently in the fields of theory development, research, practice, and education. Without something to *give order to nursing experience*, especially for the young student, it will be a chaotic event. A general concept of nursing will *identify the elements and relationships upon which the nurse should focus in nursing situations.*

Because of the complexity and continuous variability of nursing situations, Black's conceptions of "range words" and "range definitions" have value in defining nursing [9]. *Nursing* would be considered a *range word*. Individual instances of nursing would be described as constituting a range of instances, a gradual scale of embodiments grouped around some paradigms or "clear-cut" cases.

In conformity with Black, a range definition of nursing requires

1. Delineation of one or more paradigms (typical or clear-cut cases)
2. Description of a set of constitutive factors (properties of the paradigm, which may vary from instance to instance)
3. Presentation of rules for determining how, in specific instances of nursing, variations in constitutive factors determine the distance from the paradigms

In an effort to express a definition of the range word *nursing* it is appropriate to ask such questions as (1) what would be paradigms of nursing? (2) by what criteria can relative degrees of deviation from the paradigms be judged? (3) how are these criteria related? and (4) what are the presuppositions of the word *nursing*? Answering such questions should assist inquirers in the field of nursing to discover the relationships that order the set of elements comprised in the meaning of the term *nursing*. A concept of nursing expressed in this way would be complex and constitute an orderly array of elements or a system.

By concentrating on a few essentials, a general concept crystallizes the nature of a complex event in one arresting pattern. A general concept of nursing is, necessarily, a *static concept*, one that facilitates the first approach to nursing phenomena by congealing their structure in a simple pattern, representing what a number of separate entities (e.g., in nursing situations) have in common. Variations of the conceptual theme will be organized around one or more high spots — static concepts dominant enough to unite secondary concepts under the common abstraction.

In the examination of specific instances of nursing, the general, static concept of nursing becomes *dynamic*. It is seen as related to particular manifestations of nursing phenomena that will be organized around it. Upon becoming dynamic, a concept of nursing will encompass the range of a continuum of transformations, the variety of phases and appearances presented by nursing phenomena [5, pp. 178–186].

Two opposing criteria control the conceptions chosen to guide inquiry: reliability and validity [2, pp. 27–28]. Reliability requires that a concept be clear and usable, that it be free of ambiguity so that measurements or manipulations of the referents of its terms can be made precisely and repeated with uniform results. Validity requires that the substantive structure point to representative data, that it reflect as much as possible the richness and complexity of the subject matter. These two criteria oppose each other and lead to the revision of knowledge by means of research and the continuing assessment and modification of substantive structures within a discipline. Naive conceptions that enable us to begin inquiry in a complex field such as nursing lead to investigations that point to more adequate and refined conceptions of the subject matter.

A concept of nursing has concrete referents — it deals with the real world where nursing is practiced, but it frees thought and expression from the domination of that real world. If the concept is too static and oververbalized, however, it will make inadequate reference to actual nursing situations [7, pp. 138–139]. A static concept of nursing, then, must continue to become dynamic in the fields of research and practice.

A sound general concept of nursing would be a helpful instrument for integrating segments of nursing theory and relevant theory from other disciplines toward an adequate total product. In a practice discipline, a theory is a good one if adherence to it can bring about consistent, persistent, and extensive activity that in turn creates the kind of reality conceptually specified by the theory as desirable [10, pp. 433, 435]. Use of a general concept of nursing in reality situations, then, identifies those elements on which the nurse should focus, provides a base for making inferences from empirical data, and is a necessary guide in the design and production of nursing systems in society.

Different individuals, endeavoring at least tentatively to express or describe a general concept of what nursing is, may come up with different products with varying degrees of reliability and validity. Differences of opinion in ways of conceptualizing nursing phenomena are healthy *if* nurses are willing to admit that conceptions will vary in their utility and productivity and that there may be more than one good nursing theory [10, p. 433].

Concepts in a discipline vary according to their degree of productivity in generating new concepts or in holding knowledge static within the discipline. Selection of more highly valued concepts, those with a high degree of reliability and validity as a base for scientific inquiry, will result in greater productivity and should take precedence in use within the discipline. The collaboration of members of the discipline working with segments of theory and selected conceptual constructs toward a total product would best advance the structuring of nursing knowledge with economy of effort.

Selection of General Concepts of Nursing

If generalizations about what nursing is are accepted as essential guides for inquiry, nurses interested in inquiry will necessarily become involved in the task of selecting generalizations adequate for this inquiry. Selection involves a number of steps, including (1) identifying and reviewing available general concepts of nursing, (2) analyzing the concepts to isolate their component elements and the conceptualized or implicit relations among the elements, (3) measuring the analyzed concepts against criteria of adequacy, and (4) making judgments about the adequacy of each of the general concepts of nursing on the basis of results obtained from application of criteria of adequacy. These steps are preliminary to and enable the fifth step — the making of a choice. The result of the fifth step may be, for example, the choice of a developed general concept of nursing, the deferment of making a choice, or a decision that the individual or group will describe the concrete operations or events to which they will attach the term *nursing*.

The views of and convictions about nursing held by the persons involved in the selection of a general concept will affect the results obtained by them from each step of the process. In the work of identification, review, analysis, evaluation of adequacy, and final selection of a generalization about nursing, the *nursing world* of the person engaged in selection of a concept and the *nursing worlds* of the persons who invented the concepts come under the scrutiny of the selector. The selection process may involve effort toward *identification and resolution of differences* between the *nursing worlds* of the selector and the conceptualizer. The time requirements for resolution of differences may be compounded when a group of persons is involved in the selection process.

Involvement in the above-named efforts tends *to force* the selector into the role of generalizer about what nursing is. This is an essential role for every nurse who engages in nursing inquiry. The process of selection necessary for choosing a general concept of nursing thus serves two purposes: (1) decision-making relative to the concept to be adopted and (2) stimulating, or forcing, individuals to conceptualize about the reasons for and characteristics of nursing in society or, at least, confronting them with the need for such activity. The two purposes are interrelated.

Five *General Standards of Adequacy* of general concepts of nursing with subordinate statements of *criterion measures* are presented for use in determining whether there is evidence that each standard is or is not met. These standards and criterion measures are offered for consideration, evaluation, and subsequent revision through use in the steps of the selection process previously described.

GENERAL STANDARDS OF ADEQUACY

I. The general concept of nursing establishes the focus and limits of nursing in society.

  A. That which is the *object of attention* of the nurse is set forth without ambiguity.

  B. The general characteristics of *what* nurses *do* are set forth without ambiguity.

  C. The *reasons why* nurses do what they do as nurses are set forth without ambiguity.

  Note: "Without ambiguity" in A, B, and C means that nursing is clearly differentiated from other health and health-related services; linkages to specific services may or may not be explicitly stated.

  D. The end product of nursing is named. (Ultimate results such as health or wellness are not expressions of end products of nursing.)

II. The general concept of nursing sets forth the organization of nursing phenomena.

  A. *Elements* symbolized within the concept have *real-world referents.*

  B. Conceptualized *relations* among the real-world referents are explicitly stated or can be inferred from the symbolized conceptual elements.

  C. The elements and relations set forth in the statement of the concept form one or more "dominant themes" or "high spots" that can serve as organizers for the range of variation of the elements and relations.

III. The general concept of nursing has become dynamic.

  A. There is evidence of the *consistent use* of the concept by one or more persons.

  B. There is evidence that consistent use of the concept has involved *extensive activity to create reality situations* specified by the general concept.

  C. The substantive structure of the "dominant themes" of the concept is developed or under development.

  D. Isolated existing segments of nursing theory have been incorporated into the substantive structure of the dominant themes and the relations among them.

  E. There is evidence that the general concept of nursing has been used to *integrate segments of theory from other disciplines* with

    1. The broad conceptual structure of nursing

    2. The developed and developing substantive structure of the dominant themes

F. There is evidence that the efforts to make the concept dynamic have led, or are leading, to the identification and description of *useful nursing research methodologies.*

IV. The general concept of nursing exhibits reliability.
   A. General standards I and II are met.
   B. There is evidence that the concept has been used in *measuring or manipulating the referents* with precision and uniformity of results.

V. The general concept of nursing exhibits validity.
   A. There is evidence that the *substantive structure* of the *dominant themes* delineate and organize nursing data.
   B. There is evidence that the substantive structure of dominant themes has the capacity to reflect the "richness and complexity" of the *subject matter of nursing.*

The reading of the statements of standards and criteria of adequacy make it clear that evaluation of the adequacy of a general concept is a continuing process. Ideally, the process begins prior to the final selection of a general concept for use in inquiry or practice or education and continues throughout the period of use. Therefore, individuals or groups in disciplines at beginning developmental stages necessarily invent or select and use general concepts, the adequacy of which may not be demonstrated.

THE FRAME OF REFERENCE OF SCIENCE

Concept formalization and use is a continuing intellectual process as nurses develop themselves as scholars who are able to use their conceptualizations in nursing practice, research and development, or nursing education. However, the movement of nurses to develop nursing as a discipline of knowledge that has utility in practice demands that nurses become able to work within a broader and more complex frame of reference, the frame of reference of science. This places the demand on nurses to develop understanding of the character of science, how sciences advance, and the form of nursing sciences. The development of nursing sciences begins once the object of nursing and the reasons for its existence are conceptualized.

What is Science

Science seeks to provide systematic and responsibly supported explanations about objects and events in the world of human experience. Science organizes and classifies knowledge according to explanatory principles and seeks to discover and to formulate the conditions under which events occur. Science seeks to find the relations of dependence between things without regard to their bearing on existent human values [11].

Scientific knowledge is systematic. The basic framework of a science is a structure of described and conceptualized objects or events with explanations of the relationships among them. The basic framework is "filled out" as the science advances [12]. Advancement of a science results from the deliberate efforts of scientists who, as empirical inquirers, seek understanding of "data of sense" from the viewpoint of *possible relationships* among entities under investigation. Verification of insights about possible relationships continues the advancement of the sciences [12, pp. 76–78].

Explanations that constitute component parts of a science are differentiated from common-sense explanations. This differentiation is of critical importance to nurses who seek to acquire insights about nursing science. Common-sense knowledge has been contrasted with scientific knowledge by Nagel [11, pp. 1–14] and Lonergan [12, pp. 173–249]. Some points of difference between these kinds of knowledge are summarized.

1. Common sense and science operate from different viewpoints. Common sense is concerned with the concrete and particular, with mastering situations as they arise. Science is concerned with the formulation and communication of universally valid knowledge.
2. Common-sense knowledge may be accurate within some range, but the limits of its accuracy are not known and explanations of facts are not given. Science provides explanations and sets limits on its formulations.
3. Common sense is concerned with things as related to us, but science is concerned with things as related among themselves.
4. Both science and common sense reach conclusions by the self-correcting process of learning. However, the conclusions reached are different because different standards and criteria are used. Whereas

the scientist continues to ask why, the person engaged in common-sense explanations ceases to ask why as soon as it is evident that additional inquiry would not be of immediate benefit.

5. Common-sense explanations are communicated in language that is vague, indeterminant, and lacking in specificity. Scientific language is specific, determinant, abstract, and designed for use in wide-spread communication among scientists.

Stages of Development of Sciences (and Arts)

Four stages can be distinguished in the development of any science (or art). These stages are referred to as (1) natural history, (2) normative thinking, (3) science proper, and (4) application. The stages should be understood as *overlapping* and *interlocking,* not as "watertight compartments" [13].

At any stage of its development, the function of a science is to establish generalizations about the connections among empirical *events* or *objects* or their *properties.* The nature and form of the generalizations of a science will differ according to each stage of a science's development. For example, Braithwaite [14] suggests that the generalizations of a science (which he refers to as laws) in an early stage of development are those involved in classifications. Thus, classifying a system of nursing care as *wholly compensatory* [15] is to generalize that all persons in patient roles in such care systems are incapable of having an instrumental role in their self-care.

Generalizations are considered as the products of scientific endeavor. The process for arriving at and supporting generalizations combines the process of formulation of theories with the process of research (directed and controlled inquiry). The basic framework of a science and the degree to which it is filled out (i.e., advanced [12]) will determine the questions for research. The kinds of theories that are advanced to explain empirical relationships within a scientific field are associated with stages of development of a specific science. For example, "factor" theories [14, p. 53] are associated with the early stages of development of a science.

Sciences must be founded (i.e., started) by individuals. There is necessarily an *object* of *attention* and *inquiry.* Insights are attained and there is beginning understanding of the object of inquiry. Insight is the element in science that is private; it is discovery on the part of an individual engaged in inquiry. Its occurrence is both sudden and unexpected as thinking moves between the abstract and the concrete [12, pp. 3—5]. Formulated and expressed insights and theoretical systems in the early stages of development of a science are often rejected as being *nothing but* common sense. Without the formulation and expression of simple theories that represent or explain associations among things, the basic framework of a science would not be developed, for example, the expression of insights about the *reasons for* the relationships between persons in the roles of patient and nurse in health-care situations.

The Natural History Stage   In this early stage of a science's development, thinking is largely descriptive. Inquiry is directed to the question: What is the case? What is the situation? [13]. Inquiry is about events or objects as these can be viewed by the inquirer; it is not about relations among events or objects. However, a scientist selects as a focus of inquiry those events or objects that lead more directly to knowledge of relations among events or objects themselves [12, p. 292]. For example, a nursing scientist may observe and describe nurse behaviors while nurses are interacting with patients or vice versa, but the sample of nurses or patients observed may be selected with understanding of the factors that may be associated with the behaviors. Because ordinary language is not adequate for scientific description, the development of special technical terminology [12, p. 292] is started at this stage.

Stage of Normative Thinking   Inquiry in this stage is directed to the question: What ought to be the case? The norm for the object of inquiry is sought. The establishment of morphologic norms for anatomic structures and the connections among them results from this mode of thought and inquiry. Within nursing, an appropriate question for inquiry would be: How should nurses relate themselves to persons under nursing care who have no ability to control their position and movement in space? The basis for the nurse's relating of self to others who exhibit such properties would be posited in terms of some set of qualities or properties of the nurse.

The Stage of Science Proper   This is the stage of explanation, the stage when thinking and inquiry are directed to the verification of explanatory accounts of relations among events, objects, or properties thereof. Understanding of the permanent and the contingent components of the relations is sought. Four modes of explanation are utilized: deductive or classical, probabilistic or statistical, functional or teleologic, and genetic or developmental [11, pp. 21−26]. These modes of explanation should be viewed as being related rather than as operational in isolation one from the other. As expressed by Lonergan, laws derived from the statistical mode of explanation have no greater "scientific significance" than the "definitions of events" (classical formulations) whose frequencies they determine [12, p. 112].

Stage of Application   The stage of application is reached when the generalizations and explanatory systems of a science or art exhibit value in the making of predictions and prescriptions within assignable limits within the science or in another field. Prediction and prescription provide a basis for decision-making in practical affairs, including the practical affairs of research.

The Structure of Nursing Sciences
The importance for the culture of the sciences that are practice oriented has been seriously neglected by the philosophers of science. The object for study in the practical sciences is far removed from the realm of the philosopher and the natural scientist. Maritain maintains that there are sciences in the practical order and describes them to be of three types: speculatively practical, practically practical, and the knowledge of the practitioner, which is combined with the practitioner's art and is irreducible to the speculative mode [16].

Nursing is in the realm of the practical, and nursing sciences will have a practical orientation even when speculative (theoretical) in mode. Nursing sciences are grounded in the reality of deliberate human action and are limited by the object of nursing in the society. Sciences that are practice oriented seek to know not purely for the sake of knowing but for the sake of making and doing (Fig. 1-2).

It is suggested that nursing is a practical science and a set of applied sciences [13, p. 2]. A valid general theory of nursing, a theoretically practical nursing science component, provides the conceptual structure for the development of the nursing sciences. For example, the NDCG general theories of nursing and nursing system (see Chap. 5) are theoretical in mode and practical in their orientations. The conceptual structures of the two general theories provide points of theory and serve to identify types of practice problems around which the applied nursing sciences could be developed. The conceptual structures of the theories of nursing and nursing system also specify focuses for the development of the practically oriented nursing sciences. Some components of the practical nursing sciences would be generalizable to all instances of nursing. Other components would be organized by types of nursing cases in which the patient variables vary over a known range setting up requirements for different end products.

Applied science develops at the juncture between empirically identifiable elements in some subject matter and axioms or postulates or theorems derived through theoretical explanations. Its object is to derive material truth or falsity [11, pp. 220–222]. An applied science may develop as the coordinate of elements from several sciences. Applied sciences, such as engineering or medical sciences linked to practical sciences have as their object operation on a component of the concrete order, and these sciences draw from a variety of bodies of knowledge. The structure of an applied nursing science would reflect the organization of explanations and principles from one or more sciences that have utility in solving a type of problem that occurs within nursing practice situations.

Practical science (Maritain's practically practical science) is directive of action or conduct in practice situations. It is an organization of what is already known that will enable taking action toward some end product by acting in a prudential way. The structure of practical nursing science would be in the form of (1) specifications for end products (e.g., types of nursing systems to be created when certain patient factors are present), (2) diagnostic and regulatory technologies appropriate for use under specific conditions, and (3) rules of practice that would be valid and reliable directives for nurse action in all or in some types of nursing situations.

THEORY IN NURSING

Theory in nursing or any field is the result of persons offering explanations (theorizing). *Theory* is used colloquially to mean an untested idea or an opinion. Within the frame of reference of natural or applied science or the arts, *theory* is used to refer to more or less verified explanations, conceptions, or views that account for certain facts and phenomena. Theory results from the speculations of individuals about reality. It is the creative dimension of the generation of knowledge by members of disciplines. Its creation requires an intelligent and inquiring mind. The test of a theory is its utility in generating new knowledge or in the making of predictions and prescriptions in practical situations.

The development of insights about theory in nursing or other practice disciplines can be facilitated by understandings of deliberate action. Theories of action formulated and expressed by early philosophers such as Aristotle, as well as the formulations of philosophers and scientists in more recent times, provide insights about the practice dimensions of a field and at the same time express the kinds of realities that must be taken into account and understood by the practitioner and theorized about by the theorist. For example, the four levels of theory in practice disciplines proposed by Dickoff and James can be located in relation to one or more of the elements of action within situations of action.

Theory in nursing will be descriptive or explanatory of real entities that nurses encounter in their world. It will be predictive of what can or cannot be regulated or controlled through nursing. It will be predictive of stability or change in situations. And finally it will be prescriptive of actions to be performed or not performed, of means to be used, and of goals to be sought.

Theory formulation in nursing provides both a guide for practice and a basis for research. Laying out the domain and boundaries of nursing and the formalization of the proper object of nursing indicate the realities about which nurses should theorize as nurses. The acceptance of a valid and reliable general concept of nursing is a first step toward the development of momentum in the generation of nursing theories.

Nursing practice and nursing education can be advanced through more effective theory formulation in nursing. Theories to explain many of the practice operations of experienced nurses and the basis for them would contribute to nursing students' advancement in understanding and would provide frames of reference for research. To further the development of nursing as a practice discipline, there must be a merging of nursing theory with nursing research in distinct areas within nursing's domain. Only in this fashion can the applied and practical nursing sciences develop.

REFERENCES

1. Phenix, P. H. The Architectonics of Knowledge. In S. Elam (Ed.), *Education and the Structure of Knowledge.* Chicago: Rand McNally, 1964. Pp. 48–49.
2. Schwab, J. J. Structure of the Disciplines: Meanings and Significances. In G. W. Ford and L. Pugno (Eds.), *The Structure of Knowledge and the Curriculum.* Chicago: Rand McNally, 1964. Pp. 12, 25.
3. Brownowski, J. *Science and Human Values.* New York: Harper & Row, 1965. Pp. 13–14.
4. Gibson, J. Concept Learning and Concept Teaching. In R. M. Gagné and W. J. Gephart (Eds.), *Learning Research in School Subjects.* Itasca, Ill.: Peacock, 1968. P. 54.
5. Arnheim, R. *Visual Thinking.* London: Faber & Faber, 1969. Pp. 14, 54–56, 70–72.

6. Furfey, P. H. *The Scope and Method of Sociology.* New York: Harper, 1953. P. 556.
7. Gagné, R. M. *The Conditions of Learning.* New York: Holt, Rinehart & Winston, 1965. Pp. 47—51.
8. Glaser, R. Concept Learning and Concept Teaching. In R. M. Gagné and W. J. Gephart (Eds.), *Learning Research in School Subjects.* Itasca, Ill.: Peacock, 1968. P. 2.
9. Black, M. *Problems of Analysis — Philosophical Essays.* Ithaca, N.Y.: Cornell University Press, 1954. Pp. 24—29.
10. Dickoff, J., James, P., and Wiedenbach, E. Theory in a practice discipline. *Nurs. Res.* 17:415, 1968.
11. Nagel, E. *The Structure of Science.* New York: Harcourt, Brace & World, 1961. P. 10.
12. Lonergan, B. J. F. *Insight.* New York: Philosophical Library, 1957. P. 492.
13. O'Doherty, E. F. Minutes of the Meeting of the Faculty and the Committee for the Development of a Nursing Model (typewritten). The Catholic University of America, Washington, D.C., May 13, 1965. P. 2.
14. Braithwaite, R. B. *Scientific Explanation.* New York: Harper Torchbooks, 1960. Pp. 1—2, 9.
15. Orem, D. E. *Nursing Concepts of Practice.* New York: McGraw-Hill, 1971. Pp. 78—79.
16. Maritain, J. *The Degrees of Knowledge.* New York: Scribner's, 1959. Pp. 311—316, 456—459.

4

Selected Concepts of Nursing in the Public Domain

Individual nurses from the time of Florence Nightingale to the present have endeavored to conceptualize nursing or to define and express the connotation of the word *nursing*. Concepts of nursing in the public domain[1] represent incipient nursing theory, open to change and validation,[2] and serve as guides to nursing practice [1, 2]. They are illustrative of the development of nursing knowledge and as such are worthy of inquiry. What elements that are key ideas expressed in general concepts of nursing can be identified as reflections of the real world of nursing? What are the logical relationships among the elements? Do the elements and their order reveal (1) entities that are the object of nurses' attention; (2) aspects or features of the entities to which nurses attend; and (3) the way in which nurses are concerned with specific entities in certain of their aspects or features (i.e., what nursing meaning can be ascribed to them)?

A SAMPLE OF CONCEPTS

A selected sample of 14 concepts of nursing published by nurses was examined and analyzed in an effort to find answers to these questions.

Five criteria were established for selection of the sample of generalizations about nursing from the literature:

1. The statements are those of nurses educated in accord with the highest prevailing standards of the times.

---

[1] Through written publication, private experiences and ideas become public knowledge to be shared and subject to objective experiential check by others [1].

[2] A concept corresponds to a "family of conceptions." A concept is valid only if what is intended by it becomes actual (i.e., intentions are fulfilled and inquiry continues). As conceptions change, so will the concept [2].

2. The statements are published in books in contrast to articles or papers. Books were selected as the source for generalizations about nursing because it was judged that books provide greater opportunity for exposition of concepts and are most likely to be written, published, and used as the basis of education and as guides in nursing practice.

3. The books may be focused on nursing practice or on nursing education, but nursing is treated generally and not from the perspective of a specialty area, a qualifying characteristic, or a specific feature.

4. The statements expressing generalizations about nursing are those of the authors of books published in the period of modern nursing beginning with Florence Nightingale and extending to contemporary nursing.

5. The review of the literature to select books meeting the four criteria named is limited to the historical and contemporary collections of nursing works in the various libraries of four institutions, namely, the Johns Hopkins Medical Institutions, the University of Southern Mississippi, The Catholic University of America, and the National Library of Medicine.

Books were identified and a cursory examination was made for the purpose of selecting for analyses only those books that contained *explicit definitions or descriptive statements by the author characterizing the general nature of nursing.* When possible, additional published materials (in the form of journal articles) of the nurses whose concepts were analyzed were examined to identify any further development of their ideas that would clarify or amplify their concepts.

Books by 14 authors were selected. [3, 4] Publication dates span the period from 1859 to 1977. The period extending from the late 1800s through 1955 is represented in the sample by five titles. Many of the nursing books published in this period had as their focus procedures performed by nurses and descriptions of disease processes and treatment without formal statements about what nursing is.

The statements extracted from the works of an author include those expressing generalizations about what nursing is; explanatory statements to help insure correctness of im-

[3] Multiple authors are considered as one.

[4] Some well-known statements about nursing from works that do not meet the criteria for inclusion in the analyses are discussed briefly at the end of the chapter.

pressions and interpretations; and statements expressing conceptualizations about the key ideas or dominant themes of the general concept. Statements were analyzed to isolate the symbols used, the conceptualized elements and relationships, and the structure of the conceptualizations. The general approach of each author was interpreted and summarized.

The following sections include presentation of extracted statements by authors by two time periods. Expressed concepts of health and disease and of medicine are presented wherever they are explicitly related to the conceptualization of nursing. The first period, from 1859 to 1921, covers the writings of Nightingale, 1859 to 1914 [3, 4] and Shaw, 1885 to 1902 [5]. The second period begins in 1922 and ends in 1977. The works examined include those of Harmer, 1922 [6]; Frederick and Northam, 1938 [7]; Harmer revised by Henderson [8], and Henderson, 1955 to 1966 [9, 10]; Orem, 1959 to 1973 [11–13]; Abdellah, Beland, Martin, and Matheney, 1960 to 1973 [14, 15]; Orlando, 1961 to 1972 [16, 17]; Rogers, 1961 to 1970 [18, 19]; Wiedenbach, 1964 [20, 21]; Levine, 1969 to 1973 [22, 23]; King, 1971 [24]; Mitchell, 1973 to 1977 [25, 26]; and Roy, 1974 to 1976 [27, 28].

Following the presentation of extracted statements for the two time periods, a summary of each nurse's conceptualizations is presented.

EXTRACTED STATEMENTS AND SUMMARIES, 1859–1914

In 1859, *Florence Nightingale* in her book, *Notes on Nursing,* endeavored to generalize about the nature of nursing and, in the preface, related it to knowledge a layman should have.

Every woman, or at least almost every woman, in England, has, at one time or another of her life, charge of the personal health of somebody, whether child or invalid, — in other words, every woman is a nurse. Every day sanitary knowledge, or the knowledge of nursing, or in other words, of how to put the constitution in such a state as that it will have no disease, or that it can recover from disease, takes a higher place. It is recognized as the knowledge which everyone ought to have — distinct from medical knowledge, which only a profession can have [3, p. 3].

After relating nursing to health, Nightingale defined disease as follows:

... all disease, at some period or other of its course, is more or less a reparative process, not necessarily accompanied with suffering: an effort of nature to remedy a process of poisoning or of decay, which has taken place ... [3, p. 5].

Farther on she is more explicit about sanitary or good health practices:

I use the word nursing for want of a better. It has been limited to signify little more than the administration of medicines and the application of poultices. It ought to signify the proper use of fresh air, light, warmth, cleanliness, quiet, and the proper selection and administration of diet — all at the least expense of the vital power to the patient [3, p. 6].

To clarify nursing, she differentiates it from medicine as follows:

It is often thought that medicine is the curative process. It is no such thing; medicine is the surgery of functions, as surgery proper is that of limbs and organs. Neither can do anything but remove obstructions; neither can cure; nature alone cures. Surgery removes the bullet out of the limb, which is an obstruction to cure, but nature heals the wound. So it is with medicine; the function of an organ becomes obstructed; medicine so far as we know, assists nature to remove the obstruction, but does nothing more. And what nursing has to do in either case, is to put the patient in the best condition for nature to act upon him [3, pp. 74—75].

In 1893, Nightingale clearly distinguished two types of nursing, one that she named the "art of nursing proper," that is, "the art of nursing the sick," which she describes as "generally practiced by women under scientific heads — physicians and surgeons." The other she named "health nursing or general nursing," which is "the art of health, which every mother,

girl, mistress, teacher, child's nurse, every woman ought practically to learn" [4, p. 24] . Miss Nightingale identifies by
implication the knowledge that a nurse should have.

She must recognize the laws of life, the laws of health, as the nurse
proper must recognize the laws of sickness, the cause of sickness, the
symptoms of disease, or the symptoms, it may be, not of the disease,
but of the nursing, bad or good [4, p. 25] .

Given the types of nursing related to sickness and health,
Nightingale presents her concepts of health and of disease
and the relation of nursing to them.

What is sickness? Sickness or disease is nature's way of getting rid of
the effects of conditions which have interfered with health. It is nature's attempt to cure. We have to help her. Diseases are, practically
speaking, adjectives, not noun substantives. What is health? Health is
not only to be well, but to be able to use well every power we have.
What is nursing? *Both kinds of nursing are to put us in the best possible
condition for nature to restore or to preserve health — to prevent or to
cure disease or injury.* Upon nursing proper, under scientific heads,
physicians or surgeons must depend partly, perhaps mainly, whether
nature succeeds or fails in her attempts to cure by sickness. *Nursing
proper is therefore to help the patient suffering from disease to live —
just as health nursing is to keep or put the constitution of the healthy
child or human being in such a state as to have no disease.* [5]
   What is training? Training is to teach the nurse to help the patient to
live. Nursing the sick is an art, and an art requiring an organized, practical and scientific training; for nursing is the skilled servant of medicine,
surgery and hygiene. . . . The physician prescribes for supplying the
vital force, but the nurse supplies it [4, p. 26, italics added] .

Clara Weeks-Shaw was a contemporary of Nightingale. Her
concept of nursing reflects Nightingale's concept. Shaw states
that she freely used and compiled her work from available
authorities [5, p. 5]. Shaw, like Nightingale, relates nursing
to health and disease.

---

[5]Italicized passages in this and in subsequent quotations are the identified definitions of or generalizations about nursing and are signified by the notation "italics
added." Otherwise, italics are those of the author.

Health has been comprehensively defined as the "perfect circulation of pure blood in a sound organism." Any departure from either of these three conditions constitutes disease. There is recognized in nature a tendency to reparation, a predisposition to return to a condition of health, through reparation whenever there has been any deviation from them. To assist this is the object of treatment. *To keep the patient in the state most favorable for the action of this reparative tendency,* is especially the vocation of the nurse, and it is beyond a doubt those who best understand this and have the fullest acquaintance with nature's processes, will be the most successful nurses [5, p. 13, italics added].

Shaw stressed the importance of the art of nursing by saying, "in many cases, the recovery of the patient will depend more upon the care he receives than upon medical skill" [5, pp. 13–14]. She also identifies nursing activities.

Nursing properly includes, as well as the execution of the physician's orders, the administration of food and medicine, and the more personal care of the patient, attention to the condition of the sick-room, its warmth, cleanliness, and ventilation, the careful observation and reporting of symptoms, and the prevention of contagion. It is a work which falls largely, though not exclusively, to the share of women, and it has sometimes been claimed that all women make good nurses simply by virtue of their womanhood. But this is far from true . . . [5, p. 14].

Shaw continues by setting forth the attributes of the nurse and states that the patient's welfare deserves first consideration. The duties of the nurse are described as threefold: to self, to the physician, and to the patient. The nurse's duties to self are emphasized so that she can continue to help others. The duties to the physician are seen as carrying out the directives received for his prescribed measures and the duties to the patient are to do *"whatever can effect his health and comfort"* and to *"anticipate his personal wants"* [5, pp. 15–18, italics added]. Shaw emphasizes that:

. . . the relation between the nurse and patient is one of so much dependence on the one side, and so much helpfulness on the other, as to tend to develop what may be described as the maternity of nursing. A sick person is, for the time being, as a child, and looks to his nurse for a mother's care [5, p. 19].

In describing the nurse—patient relationship, at the end of her first chapter, Shaw recognizes differences between the home nurse and the hospital nurse [5, pp. 22—23].

Summaries of Extracted Statements

Summaries of the Nightingale[6] and Shaw approaches follow. Summaries are presented in the form of descriptive statements, without reference to time of publication when statements from more than one book are interpreted and summarized.

Logical consistency and a unified conceptual product characterize *Nightingale's* approach to generalizing about nursing. Her approach is summarized in the statements that follow.

1. Nursing is knowledge the lay person should have. It is "sanitary knowledge" or knowledge of "how to put the constitution" or "the patient in the best condition for nature to act."
2. The denotation of the term *nursing* is extended beyond the common usage of the time to include hygienic care of individuals and their environment.
3. Two types of nursing are distinguished and symbols attached to each — health or general nursing, and nursing the sick or nursing proper. The two types of nursing are conceptualized as having a common general purpose and each type as having a specific purpose; the condition that nursing should conserve "the vital power" of the patient is specified.
4. The proper object of nursing is differentiated from that of medicine on the basis of differences of functions and results.
5. Regulation of the condition of the patient and his environment as a function of nursing is expressed in words such as "put" and "the proper use" of hygienic measures.
6. Preventive health care is identified as an explicit function in nursing.
7. The effects and results of nursing are described in terms of "the best condition for nature to act" and "at the least expense" to the patient's "vital power."

[6]It should be noted that Nightingale's works were published prior to and after Shaw's book. Nightingale's 1914 work was posthumous.

8. Nursing is related to the branches of medicine with the specification that the goal of nursing is the same regardless of the form of treatment received by patients — medical or surgical.

9. Physicians and surgeons are specified as "partly" to "mainly" dependent upon nursing proper for "nature's" success or failure in "her attempts to cure by sickness." No general health-care role is ascribed to medicine.

10. The practitioner of general or health nursing is described as anyone who has responsibility for the health of another; the practitioner of health nursing is differentiated from the practitioner of sick nursing or nursing proper who is prepared by specialized training and practices in relationship to physicians.

11. Nursing is conceptualized as an art and as a body of knowledge. Knowledge required for general or health nursing is described as sanitary knowledge or hygiene. Knowledge essential for nursing the sick includes medicine, surgery, and hygiene.

12. Knowledge that nurses should have is specified as including knowledge of the effects and results of nursing "bad or good."

The conceptualizations of *Shaw* reflect those of Nightingale, particularly those that express the purpose of nursing. Innovations and developments include her conceptualization of the nurse—patient relationship, extension of nursing functions, and introduction of symbols.

1. The functions of nursing are extended to include "prevention of contagion" and anticipation of the personal wants of the patient.

2. Aspects of hygienic care are symbolized as "more personal care of the patient."

3. The patient's welfare is described as the first consideration of the nurse, but duties of the nurse to self and physician are specified.

4. The helping-dependency relationship between nurse and patient is made explicit and symbolized by the term "the maternity of nursing."

5. The proper object of nursing is differentiated from that of medicine on the basis of differences of functions and results.

6. The recovery of the patient in some instances is said to be more dependent on nursing than on medical skill.

7. Nurses are named by place of practice — the home nurse and the hospital nurse.

8. Nursing is conceptualized as an art but success in nursing is attributed to (a) having full acquaintance with nature's processes and (b) understanding the purpose of nursing.

EXTRACTED STATEMENTS AND SUMMARIES, 1922—1977

Bertha Harmer in her 1922 *Text-Book of the Principles and Practice of Nursing* takes a broad social perspective on nursing and describes "The Object of Nursing, What It Is, and What It Includes" as follows:

Nursing is rooted in the needs of humanity and is founded on the ideal of service. *Its object is not only to cure the sick and heal the wounded but to bring health and ease, rest and comfort to mind and body, to shelter, nourish, and protect and to minister to all those who are helpless or handicapped, young, aged or immature. Its object is to prevent disease and to preserve health.* Nursing is, therefore, linked with every other social agency which strives for the prevention of disease and the preservation of health. The nurse finds herself not only concerned with the care of the individual but with the health of a people [6, p. 3, italics added].

Harmer, like Shaw, emphasizes Nightingale's notions of nursing. Her listing of nursing activities [6, p. 4] includes: "care of the patient's surroundings (which should be clean, attractive, quiet, orderly, and comfortable) and all of the things which add to his welfare and promote his recovery"; "personal care of the patient — bathing, feeding, making comfortable and attending to his personal wants, mental or physical"; assistance to the physician — "preparing for and assisting with examinations, treatments, operations and tests, and observing and reporting the condition of the patient and results of treatments, etc."; and "administration of special diets, drugs and treatments, etc., ordered."

Harmer also included as nursing functions [6, p. 4]:

1. Provision of teaching for nurses and patients in hospitals — "the older nurses teach the younger nurses and each nurse consciously or unconsciously by example teaches the patients, especially the children, the standards of personal hygiene."
2. "Informing the patients that, in the hospital, there is a social service department which exists in order that patients, in need of its care, may consult with it and be relieved of financial difficulties and of worries regarding conditions in their homes" [6, p. 4].

In relation to teaching, Harmer goes on to note that the problems in public health work are approached on an educational basis, "teaching the individual proper habits of living relating to food, rest, exercise, recreation, sleep and all the conditions which insure health of body and mind and increased resistance to disease" [6, p. 4].

Hester Frederick and Ethel Northam, in 1938, describe nursing as an art founded in service, stating that:

It requires the application of scientific knowledge and nursing skills and affords opportunities for *constructive work in the care and relief of patients and their families. . . .* Modern nursing is by no means limited to the *giving of expert physical care to the sick,* important as this is. It is more far reaching, including as it does *helping the patient to adjust to unalterable situations,* such as personal, family and economic conditions, *teaching him and others in the home and in the community to care for themselves, guiding him in the prevention of illness through hygienic living, and helping him to use the available community resources to these ends* [7, p. 3, italics added].

Virginia Henderson's definition of nursing, which is internationally recognized, was published in 1955 in the fifth edition of the *Textbook of the Principles and Practice of Nursing* (her revision of Harmer).

Nursing is primarily assisting the individual (sick or well) in the performance of those activities contributing to health, or its recovery (or to a peaceful death) that he would perform unaided if he had the necessary strength, will, or knowledge. It is likewise the unique contribution of nursing to help the individual to be independent of such assistance as soon as possible [8, p. 4].

According to Henderson, in this defined area of health care, the nurse is the expert and can initiate and control activities. This includes helping the patient to carry out the physician's therapeutic plan. All persons on the health-care team serve to assist the patient, who is the central figure. The unique function of the nurse is to serve as substitute for what the patient lacks to make him "complete," "whole," or "independent" with respect to physical strength, will, or knowledge to reach good health [8, pp. 4—5]. The primary responsibility of the nurse is seen to be that of helping the patient with his daily pattern of living or with those health-related activities he ordinarily performs without assistance [8, p. 5].

In Henderson's later books, *ICN Basic Principles of Nursing Care,* 1960 [9, p. 5], and *The Nature of Nursing,* 1966 [10, p. 15], revisions of the 1955 definitions are made but the essential ideas are unchanged.[7] The definition presented in *The Nature of Nursing* is adapted to focus upon "the unique function of the nurse" and is represented by Henderson as "the crystallization of my ideas" [10, p. 15]. In both the 1960 and 1966 books, Henderson describes 14 "components of basic nursing" [9, pp. 9—10] or "basic nursing care" [10, pp. 16—17] based on patient hygienic needs and needs for healthful living. Henderson contends that the nurse is the authority on basic nursing care, that is, helping the patient with these 14 types of activities or providing conditions to make it possible for the patient to perform them unaided. The 14 components of basic nursing are the basis for independent nursing practice, according to Henderson. Diagnosing, prescribing treatment for disease, and making a prognosis are seen as the physician's functions. The nurse may have to assume some of them under certain circumstances [10, pp. 16—17, 30].

Dorothea Orem's concept of nursing was first published in 1959.

Nursing is perhaps best *described as the giving of direct assistance to a person, as required, because of the person's specific inabilities in self-care resulting from a situation of personal health.* Care as required may be continuous or periodic. Self-care means the care which all persons require each day. It is the personal care which adults give to themselves, including attention to ordinary health requirements, and the following of the medical directives of their physicians. Nursing may be required

---

[7] The definition is not essentially changed in the latest edition of *The Principles and Practice of Nursing,* 6th ed., by Virginia Henderson and Gladys Nite, New York: Macmillan, 1978, pp. 14, 22, 34—36.

by persons in any age group, but it is the situation of health and not the dependencies arising from age which initiates requirements for nursing. Requirements for nursing are modified and eventually eliminated when there is progressive favorable change in the state of health of the individual, or when he learns to be self-directing in daily self-care [11, pp. 5−6, italics added].

In her 1971 book, *Nursing: Concepts of Practice,*[8] Orem describes how and why nursing is different from other health services:

Every human service has a special concern for some aspect of human functioning or daily living which defines what the service does and, thus, differentiates it from other services. Nursing has as its special concern *man's need for self-care action and the provision and management of it on a continuous basis in order to sustain life and health, recover from disease or injury, and cope with their effects.* . . .

The condition which validates the existence of a requirement for nursing in an adult *is the absence of the ability to maintain for himself continuously that amount and quality of self-care which is therapeutic in sustaining life and health, in recovering from disease or injury, or in coping with their effects.* With children, the condition is the *inability of the parent (or guardian)* to maintain continuously for the child that amount and quality of care which is therapeutic. Therapeutic is used to mean supportive of life processes, remedial or curative as related to malfunction due to disease processes, as well as contributory to personal development and maturing [12, pp. 1−2].[9]

Nursing is described as "a personal, family, and community service within the health field" [12, p. 41]. The focus of nursing for individuals is differentiated from that of medicine, and the roles and relationships of the patient, nurse, and physician are described and articulated with roles of other health workers [12, pp. 46, 49−50].

Orem develops and expresses concepts underlying two main conceptual elements — self-care and self-care inabilities or limitations — contained within her generalizations about

[8]In 1968, copies of this book in manuscript form were distributed for review and validation in nursing education and practice situations.

[9]From *Nursing: Concepts of Practice* by Dorothea E. Orem. Copyright © 1971 by McGraw-Hill, Inc. Used with permission of McGraw-Hill Book Co.

what nursing is. Two types of self-care, universal and health-deviation self-care, and self-care limitations are described in the 1959 book [11, pp. 48–62] and are further developed in the 1971 publication [12, pp. 13–36]. Both elements are used in describing types of nursing situations or nursing cases and also in expressing a concept of nursing as an art [12, p. 47].

The goals of nursing and criterion measures of nursing effectiveness are developed around the accomplishment of self-care of a therapeutic quality and around the role of the patient or others in its accomplishment.

For activities to be considered in the realm of nursing, they must be consciously selected and directed by the nurse toward accomplishing nursing goals within a health care situation. On this basis, *the results that nurses achieve through their nursing acts are beneficial to patients to the degree that (1) the patient's self-care is accomplished; (2) the nursing actions are helpful in moving the patient toward responsible action in matters of self-care (the patient may move toward steadily increasing independence or adapt to interruptions in the exercise of his capacities or to steadily declining capacities for self-care action); or (3) members of the patient's family or a non-nurse who attends the patient becomes increasingly competent in making decisions relative to the continuing daily personalized care of the patient or in providing and managing the patient's care using nurse supervision and consultation as required. One or all of these general goals of nursing action may be appropriate in specific nursing situations* [12, p. 156, italics added].[10]

The nursing process is described in relation to the object of nursing and nursing goals [12, p. 157]. To determine why a patient needs nursing, Orem specifies that the nurse should seek information about six factors, which together constitute a nursing focus. These are:

... the patient's health state, the physician's perspective of the patient's health situation, the patient's perspective of his health situation, the health results sought for the patient and their relationship to the patient's life, health, and his effective living, the patient's requirements for therapeutic self-care, and the patient's abilities and inabilities to perform therapeutic self-care [12, p. 159].[10]

[10] From *Nursing: Concepts of Practice* by Dorothea E. Orem. Copyright © 1971 by McGraw-Hill, Inc. Used with permission of McGraw-Hill Book Co.

Three types of nursing systems, the wholly compensatory, the partly compensatory, and the supportive-developmental systems, are described. The type of nursing system results from the nurse's selection and use of methods of nursing assistance which serve to delineate the roles of both the patient and nurse [12, pp. 77—81]. Five general methods of assisting applicable to a variety of nursing situations are described in some detail [12, pp. 72—77].

A further development of Orem's concept in terms of nursing systems was published in the first edition of this book in 1973 [13, pp. 67—91; see Chap. 5 of this edition].

Faye Abdellah, Irene Beland, Almeda Martin, and Ruth Matheney, in a joint work in 1960 defined nursing [14] and reaffirmed it as "unchanged" in 1973 [15, p. 18].

Nursing is a service to individuals and to families; therefore, to society. It is based upon an art and science which mold the attitudes, intellectual competencies, and technical skills of the individual nurse into the desire and ability to help people, sick or well, cope with their health needs, and may be carried out under general or specific medical direction [14, p. 24, italics added].

Nursing as a service involves:

. . . (1) recognizing the nursing problems of the patient; (2) deciding the appropriate course of action to take in terms of relevant nursing principles; (3) providing continuous care of the individual's total health needs; (4) providing continuous care to relieve pain and discomfort and provide immediate security for the individual; (5) adjusting the total nursing care plan to meet the patient's individual needs; (6) helping the individual to become more self-directing in attaining or maintaining a healthy state of mind and body; (7) instructing nursing personnel and family to help the individual do for himself that which he can within his limitations; (8) helping the individual to adjust to his limitations and emotional problems; (9) working with allied health professions in planning for optimum health on local, state, national, and international levels; and (10) carrying out continuous evaluation and research to improve nursing techniques and to develop new techniques to meet the health needs of people [14, p. 25].

Five elements of nursing practice are described. Briefly, they include (1) human relations skills; (2) observation and communication in reporting signs and symptoms and deviations from normal behavior; (3) interpretation of observations to identify deviations from health as nursing problems; (4) analysis of the nursing problem and selection of appropriate nursing actions; and (5) organization of the nurse's effort to achieve nursing results by helping "the patient to return to health or what can be approximate normal health for him" [14, p. 26].

Twenty-one nursing problems derived from the patient's needs are identified [14, pp. 16—17]. The typology of nursing problems to be solved is described as having a focus "on the physical, biological, social-psychological needs of the patient and provides a more meaningful basis for organization than the categories of systems of the body" [14, p. 27]. The need for development of a typology of nursing treatments for the identified nursing problems is also recognized [14, pp. 17—19].

Ida Jean Orlando, in *The Dynamic Nurse—Patient Relationship* published in 1961, states that *"any individual nurses another when he carries, in whole or in part, the burden of responsibility for what the person cannot yet or can no longer do alone"* [16, p. 5, italics added]. The responsibility of nursing is seen as different from that of medicine, which is described as "responsible for prevention and treatment of disease." Nursing *"offers whatever help the patient may require for his needs to be met* (italics added), *i.e., for his physical and mental comfort to be assured as far as possible while he is undergoing some form of medical treatment or supervision"* [16, p. 5].

A "deliberative nursing process" is described. The nurse initiates systematic action to ascertain the patient's immediate need before acting to meet the need [16, p. 90]. The book is an outgrowth of a project to integrate mental health principles in a basic nursing curriculum and is based on a synthesis of the author's own experience [16, pp. vi and ix].

Orlando's concept of nursing provided a basis for a nursing service study conducted in a psychiatric hospital in 1972. "The function of professional nursing is conceptualized as finding out and meeting the patient's immediate needs for help" [17, p. 20]. Nursing "is concerned with providing direct assistance to individuals in whatever setting . . . for the purpose of avoiding, relieving, diminishing or curing the individual's sense of helplessness" [17, p. 12]. The product of nursing activity is described as " 'improvement' in the patient's immediate behavior . . ." [17, p. 22]. "This observable change" indicates to the nurse whether "her activity relieved, prevented or diminished the patient's sense of helplessness" [17, p. 21]. The "deliberative nursing process" is redefined as the "nursing process discipline," a series of acts which both nurse and patient go through [17, pp. 24—27].

Martha Rogers expressed a concept of nursing in a 1961 publication [18, p. 23]. The object of nursing was presented in terms of the movement of man toward maximum health.

In her 1970 book, Rogers says that "the concern of nursing is with man in his entirety, his wholeness. Nursing's body of scientific knowledge seeks to describe, explain, and predict about human beings" [19, p. 3] and is derived from "the life process in man" [19, p. 96].

She states that:

Nursing aims to assist people in achieving their maximum health potential. Maintenance and promotion of health, prevention of disease, nursing diagnosis, intervention, and rehabilitation encompass the scope of nursing's goals [19, p. 86, italics added].

The social role of nursing is stated. "Nursing exists to serve people. Its direct and overriding responsibility is to society. Nursing has no dependent functions but, like all professions, it has many collaborative ones" [19, p. 122].

Rogers says that "nursing judgments and actions are not predicated upon disease entities, nor do they have their central focus on subsystem pathology" [19, p. 124]. Finally, Rogers makes the statement:

Professional practice in nursing seeks to promote symphonic interaction between man and environment, to strengthen the coherence and integrity of the human field, and to direct and redirect patterning of the human and environmental fields for realization of maximum health potential [19, p. 122, italics added].

Ernestine Wiedenbach, in 1964, on the basis of 40 years of experience [20, p. vii], published her statement of the purpose of clinical nursing:

. . . to facilitate the efforts of the individual to overcome the obstacles which currently interfere with his ability to respond capably to demands made of him by his condition, environment, situation and time [20, pp. 14–15, italics added].

In essence, the nurse seeks "to meet the need the individual is experiencing as a need-for-help" [20, p. 15]. Wiedenbach, like Orlando, conceives of nursing as deliberative action. Wiedenbach specifies four components of nursing practice: (1) *"identification* of the patient's experienced need-for-help"; (2) *"ministration* of the help needed"; (3) *"validation* that the help provided was indeed the help needed"; and (4) the indirect component of *"coordination of resources for help and of help provided,"* which has three functional elements — *"reporting, consulting,* and *conferring"* [20, p. 31]. In a 1970 journal article [21], Wiedenbach describes nursing as a practice discipline involving goal-directed action and revises her statement of the purpose of nursing.

Myra Estrin Levine describes nursing as human interaction, ". . . a discipline rooted *in the organic dependency of the individual human being on his relationships with other human beings"* [22, p. 1, italics added]. Nursing also is described as intervention to support and promote the patient's adaptation.

The nurse participates actively in every patient's environment and much of what she does supports his adaptations as he struggles in the predicament of illness. Nursing intervention means that the nurse interposes her skill and knowledge into the course of events that affects the patient. Thus, nursing intervention must be founded not only on scientific

*knowledge but specifically on recognition of the individual's organismic
response which indicates the nature of the adaptation taking place. . . .*

When *nursing intervention influences the adaptation favorably, or toward renewed social well-being,* then the nurse is acting in a *therapeutic
sense. When the nursing intervention cannot alter the course of the
adaptation* — when her best efforts can only maintain the status quo or
fail to halt a downward course — then the nurse is acting in a *supportive
sense* [22, p. 10, italics added].

Nursing principles are said to be "conservation" principles
based on the organismic nature of the human response to the
environment. Conservation is described as "to keep together,"
that is, to "maintain a proper balance between active nursing
intervention coupled with patient participation on the one
hand and the safe limits of the patient's ability to participate
on the other" [22, pp. 10–11]. Nursing intervention is described in relation to four conservation principles of nursing,
namely, conservation of energy, structural integrity, personal
integrity, and social integrity [22, p. 11].

"The four conservation principles have as a postulate the
unity and integrity of the individual, recognizing that every
response to every environmental stimulus results from the
integrated and unified nature of the human organism" [22,
p. 11].

In the 1973 second edition of her work, Levine indicates
that the "whole man" is the focus of nursing intervention
[23, p. vii]. The concept of nursing is unchanged. The word
"holistic" is substituted [23, p. 13] for the word "organismic" used in the earlier definition [22, p. 10].

Imogene King explored the dimensions of nursing and
proposed a "conceptual frame of reference for professional
nursing" [24, p. 2] in 1971. According to King, *"Generally,
the basic abstraction of nursing is the phenomenon of man
and his world"* [24, p. 11]. One approach to dealing with
"this complexity" suggested by King, "is to identify specific
goals for nursing care to determine ways that individuals and
groups cope with health and illness and adapt to changes in
health states" [24, p. 11].

Four universal ideas — social systems, health, perception, and interpersonal relations — need exploration, King says, "as sources of the conceptual base of the dimensions of nursing, that is, the physical, emotional, social, and intellectual state and capacity of individuals and groups encountered by nurses" [24, p. 21]. Selection of these concepts was based upon King's belief about nursing:

. . . nurses, in the performance of their roles and responsibilities, assist individuals and groups in society to attain, maintain, and restore health. In the process of functioning in social institutions, nurses assist individuals to meet their basic needs at some point in time in the life cycle when they cannot do this for themselves. An understanding of basic human needs in the physical, social, emotional, and intellectual realm of the life process from conception to old age, within the context of social systems of the culture in which nurses live and work, is essential and basic content for learning the practice of nursing [24, p. 22].

The dynamics of her frame of reference are described as follows:

Man functions in *social systems* through *interpersonal relationships* in terms of his *perceptions* which influence his life and *health*. The framework is social systems; the methods are interpersonal relationships; and the determinants are perception and health [24, p. 22].

The goal of nursing is to help individuals and groups attain, maintain, and restore health. One means to achieve the goal is nursing care. In nursing situations where the goal of life and health cannot be achieved, as in a terminal illness, nurses give care and help individuals die with dignity [24, p. 84].

After describing her frame of reference, King gives her definition of nursing:

NURSING IS A PROCESS OF ACTION, REACTION, INTERACTION, AND TRANSACTION, WHEREBY NURSES ASSIST INDIVIDUALS OF ANY AGE AND SOCIOECONOMIC GROUP TO MEET THEIR BASIC NEEDS IN PERFORMING ACTIVITIES OF DAILY LIVING AND TO COPE WITH HEALTH AND ILLNESS AT SOME PARTICULAR POINT IN THE LIFE CYCLE [24, p. 89, italics added].

The elements of the process model are conceptualized as involving perception, judgment, action leading to reaction (verbal and nonverbal), interaction, and transaction relative to both patient and nurse in the achievement of the goals of health or adjustment to health problems [24, p. 126]. Finally, "The specific function of nursing is assistance to individuals to help them cope with a health problem or adjust to interference in their health state" [24, p. 126].

Pamela H. Mitchell published a definition of nursing in 1973. In the introductory passages of her book, nursing is defined:

Nursing is a means to help people whose actual or potential deviations from health have impaired their ability to cope with some aspects of daily living. Nursing care may be aimed at preventing the initial or further deviations from health, at restoring or enhancing the ability to cope with daily activity, and at maintaining or sustaining the person's capacities through a health problem. These services may be provided independently of other health professions or in collaboration with them [25, p. vii, italics added].

In the 1977 revision of her book, Mitchell adds the following statement to her definition of nursing: ". . . nursing seeks to help persons whose response to problems of daily living actually or potentially alters their health" [26, p. ix].

The focus of nursing was stated as ". . . *helping people cope with those difficulties in daily living which are associated with their actual or potential health/illness problems or the treatment thereof.* Orem calls this ability to cope with daily living, 'self-care' (1971)" [25, p. 28]. [11] In 1977 two notions were added to the original delineation of the nursing focus. These were to help people to "respond positively to" their difficulties in daily living and to "dying" [26, p. 26].

[11] Orem defines self-care as an action system that is but one component of daily living [12, pp. 1, 15]. Orem's definition is as follows: "Self-care is the practice of activities that individuals personally initiate and perform on their own behalf in maintaining life, health and well-being. . . . Self-care is an adult's personal, continuous contribution to his own health and well-being" [12, p. 13].

The focus of nursing is differentiated from medicine in that the physician is described as being primarily concerned with "determining and removing the cause or in treating the health/illness problem, and only secondarily with the person's daily functioning during the course of it. Nurses have an interdependent role with physicians in the therapy of a disability or illness, but they have a primary role in helping the person live with or avoid further disability, and in promoting wellness — living to one's fullest capacities" [25, p. 28].

"The general goals of nursing are to prevent disability and to restore, maintain, or rehabilitate ability" [25, pp. 75–76]. Diagnosis of nursing problems is concerned with estimates of "functional disability" which are determined by "analyzing the patient–client's status in terms of normative standards, i.e., what the 'healthy' or 'normal' person should be able to do" [25, p. 74].

Mitchell states that nursing is "an applied field, using concepts from the natural, physical, and behavioral sciences and concepts from medical practice to derive principles for action" [25, pp. 72–73].

Sister Callista Roy's nursing model appears in a chapter of a 1974 book on conceptual models for nursing practice. Roy's model served as a basis for her 1976 introductory nursing textbook. In the 1974 work, nursing was defined in relation to its goal:

All nursing activity will be aimed at promoting man's adaptation in his physiologic needs, his self-concept, his role function, and his interdependence relations during health and illness [27, p. 139, italics added].

The four adaptive modes, or ways, of acting specified in the statement were identified by Roy from a survey of 500 samples of patient behaviors [27, p. 138]. Roy specifies the goal of nursing as man's adaptations in the four named modes. Roy cites four reasons why nursing's goal should be sought. Reasons are viewed as values inherent in the goal. These are expressed in terms of social significance, meaning for patient welfare, conservation of patient energy, and types of stimuli to which patient as person adapts [27, p. 139].

Nursing assessment is said to require "identification of patient behaviors in each of the adaptive modes" and "the focal, contextual, and residual factors influencing the behavior" [27, p. 141]. Nursing interventions aim to support and promote man's adaptation [27, p. 139]. This is done by manipulating the influencing factors — the focal, contextual, and residual stimuli [28, pp. 141–142]. Nursing goals are stated as behavioral outcomes [28, p. 19]. Adaptive responses, as goals, are a set of behaviors that "maintains the integrity of the individual" [28, p. 13].

In her 1976 work, Roy restated the goal of nursing as follows:

> . . . to promote man's adaptation in each of the adaptive modes in situations of health and illness. The states of varying degrees of health or illness can be represented by a continuous line called the health-illness continuum . . . Adaptation problems have been defined as situations resulting from inadequate responses to meet need deficits or excesses. As man moves along the continuum between maximum wellness and maximum illness, he will encounter adaptation problems. These problems are the concern of the nurse. Her goal will be to solve the problem and bring about adaptation [28, p. 18].

Summaries of Extracted Statements

Nurses' approaches to conceptualizing about nursing during the period 1922 to 1977 are summarized. The summaries are based on the extracted statements.

The conceptual systems of Nightingale and Shaw seem to be reflected in *Harmer's* generalizations. However, the operations of "nature" are no longer explicit within statements of the "object" of nursing. The purpose of nursing now is stated in relation to (1) categories of recipients — sick and wounded; helpless or handicapped; young, aged, or immature; and (2) results desirable for, or actions needed by, recipients by categories.

Harmer includes the notion of physical and mental health
in her conceptual system and emphasizes promotion of health
and prevention of disease. She makes explicit references to
ways of helping hospitalized patients by teaching them hygiene
and informing them about available social services. Nurses are
categorized by place of practice, and nursing activities related
to the physician's work are identified. Nursing now is linked
to social agencies in the health field, not just to medicine. The
public health work of nurses is represented as primarily educational and as having a focus on hygienic practices.

Harmer makes explicit the notion that nursing has its
"roots" or foundations in *people* — in their needs and the
ideal of service for others.

Frederick and Northam generalize about the practice of
nursing with an emphasis on functions. They explicitly extend
the object of nursing to include *families of patients,* and
functions of nursing to include helping patients to adjust to
unalterable situations and to use community resources. A number of ways of helping patients are expressed: giving care to,
teaching, guiding, and helping in use of resources. Patients
and others are characterized as *care agents.*

Frederick and Northam contribute new conceptualizations,
continuing, however, within the conceptual system of Nightingale, Shaw, and Harmer.

A concisely stated definition conveying the connotations
of nursing is one of *Virginia Henderson's* contributions to
concept formalization in nursing. The concept is expressed in
ordinary language and in relation to reality elements. Her
definition initiates the movement away from conceptualizing
the object of nursing in terms of the "constitution" or "nature's" operations or the specifics of curing, healing, or preventing as related to disease.

The object of nursing is expressed as a duality — activities
individuals "usually" perform and reasons why they cannot
perform them. "Usually" is interpreted as a boundary-setting

term. Results of nursing are extended beyond those already identified to include a peaceful death and independence of nursing assistance as soon as possible. Individuals are conceptualized as health-care agents and nursing as activity in the form of assisting.

Henderson introduces the terms "basic nursing care" and "independent nursing practice" and relates the two. One of the elements of the concept — activities ordinarily performed by individuals — is developed in the form of a listing of activities.

Generalizations about nursing formulated by *Orem* are developed in relation to individuals. The proper object of nursing is expressed in terms of inabilities of individuals to engage in self-care because of health or health-related reasons. Nursing is conceptualized as action, as assistance. Results of nursing are specified in relation to self-care and self-care agency of individuals. Orem's general concept of nursing corresponds in substance to that of Henderson. Differences are in the symbolization used and in the manner of expressing boundaries.

Orem's efforts have resulted in a conceptual system in which there is a development of the substantive structure of each of the conceptual elements comprising the general concept. Symbolization is introduced and terms are defined. States of health and illness are admitted into the conceptual system through the conceptual elements — self-care and health-derived or health-related self-care limitations. Orem continues the movement away from expressing the formal object of nursing in terms of the constitution or nature's operations or health or disease.

Abdellah, Beland, Martin, and Matheney express generalizations about nursing in terms of attributes of the nurse and a continuation of the dependency theme. Recipients of nursing are characterized as "sick or well," requiring assistance to cope with health problems derived from "physical, biological, or social-psychological needs" such as "pain and discomfort," "insecurity," and inability to become "self-directing in attaining and maintaining health." Elements of nursing practice are described in terms of a problem-solving process, the results of which are to help the individual to "return to health or what can be approximate normal health for him." Nursing "may be carried out" under medical direction.

The focus of *Orlando's* conceptualizations is identified as the individual who nurses. Nursing from this viewpoint is conceptualized as being responsible for what others cannot do alone and determining the immediate need for help. Results of nursing are: *needs met, physical and mental comfort,* and *relief of the sense of helplessness.* Recipients of nursing are described as under medical care or supervision.

Orlando continues to develop the helpfulness-dependency relationship of nurse and patient, which was made explicit by Shaw. Nursing is viewed as deliberate action in interpersonal situations and symbolized as a "deliberative nursing process" or "the nursing process discipline."

Generalizing about nursing is approached in an eclectic fashion by *Rogers.* There are statements about (1) what nursing aims to do, (2) nursing's goals, and (3) what professional practice in nursing seeks. The first is expressed in terms of assisting people in the achievement by them of their maximum health potential; the second, in terms of (a) results specific for states of health and disease, (b) results of and steps of the nursing process, and (c) the process of rehabilitation; the third, in terms of (a) interaction of man and environment and (b) the human and environmental fields and their patterning in relation to "realization of maximum health potential."

Rogers places nursing in a social context, viewing nursing as a service to society and as a body of scientific knowledge.

Wiedenbach expresses generalizations about nursing in relation to the recipient of nursing and the nurse. Recipients are conceptualized as agents overcoming obstacles and experiencing needs for help. Obstacles are identified as those that prevent the agent from meeting demands arising from "his condition, environment, situation, and time." Health and disease and health-care practices or processes are not mentioned in the definition, but they can be inferred from the named sources of demands on the patient.

Generalizations about nursing are expressed by *Levine* in relation to ill patients in environments (of which nurses are parts) adapting and revealing their adaptations through holistic responses. The nurse is viewed as an agent in the patient's environment who "interposes" skill and knowledge into the "course of events" affecting the patient. Nursing is conceptualized as "human interaction" and is viewed as a discipline with its foundations in the dependency of individuals on other individuals in human societies and on four conservation principles of nursing.

King takes a process focus in generalizing about nursing. Process subsumes action, reaction, interaction, and transaction. Process is identified as the means nurses use to assist individuals. Individuals are described as being of any age, any socioeconomic group, and at some particular point in the life cycle. Assistance is concerned with meeting "basic needs in performing activities of daily living" and "coping with health and illness."

Mitchell expresses the object of nursing attention as a duality — a focus on patient health state and patient agency in daily living. Results of nursing actions are described from these two views. One is focused upon preventing "deviations from health" and the other upon assisting people by "restoring or enhancing" their "ability to cope with daily activity" and by "maintaining or sustaining" a "person's capacities through a health problem."

Roy's generalizations about nursing are developed in terms of human adaptation. The object of nursing is expressed as the goal of promoting "man's adaptation" in health and illness in four identified modes. Results of nursing are identified as the adaptive responses that "maintain the integrity of the individual" in four areas — "physiologic needs," "self-concept," "role function," and "interdependence relations." Nursing actions involve assessment of patient behaviors and manipulation of factors that influence adaptation levels in these four modes.

ANALYSIS OF THE CONCEPTUALIZATIONS

The statements of the general concepts of nursing as identified by the NDCG were analyzed to identify the appearance and subsequent development of key ideas. Nightingale's generalizations were utilized as the base for identifying change. The results of this analysis are presented in Figures 4-1 through 4-14.

The series of diagrams indicates (1) the ways of expressing that which is the concern, or the specific object, of attention of nurses, and (2) the appearance of dominant themes, including relations among them. These diagrams also aid in placing the general concepts of nursing in categories using the structure of the concept as the organizing principle. For example, the *patient—nurse dependency relationship* made explicit by Shaw is evident in subsequent concepts to greater or lesser degrees; and the identification of recipients of nursing as *health-care (self-care) agents* implicit in the Frederick and Northam listing of ways of helping patients is developed explicitly in the concepts of Henderson, Orem, Abdellah et al., Orlando, Wiedenbach, Mitchell, and King.

Another analysis was done to identify commonalities and differences among the expressed general concepts. Three commonalities were noted and many differences.

Commonalities included the ideas that (1) nursing is result-producing activity that involves nurses in helping relationships with recipients of nursing; (2) nursing is a unique service, an entity because of its own proper activities and, therefore, distinct from medicine; and (3) nursing is related to the state of health or well-being, or the absence thereof, in recipients of nursing. These ideas, while common to all the general concepts, were not always explicitly expressed. For example, in Nightingale the condition of the recipient's health is an element of the concept, in Orem it is subsumed within the structure of an element, and in Wiedenbach it can be inferred from an element.

Differences in the statements of general concepts were clustered around ways of symbolizing recipients of nursing, the forms of nursing as action, and the results of nursing.

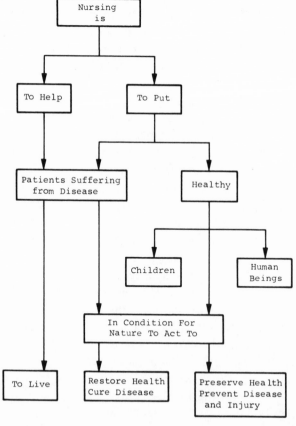

Figure 4-1 Dominant themes in Nightingale's concept of nursing; the formalization of health and disease themes.

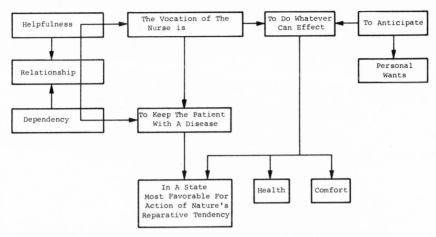

Figure 4-2   Dominant themes in Shaw's concept of nursing; emergence of the personal and interpersonal themes.

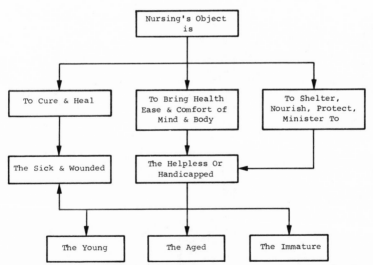

Figure 4-3   Dominant themes in Harmer's concept of nursing; development of the patient dependency theme.

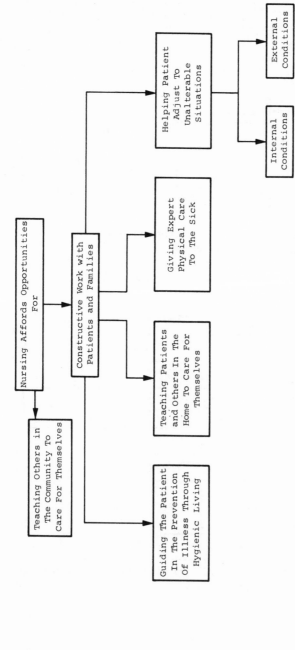

Figure 4-4 Dominant themes in Frederick and Northam's concept of nursing; emergence of patient agency theme and of ways to promote agency.

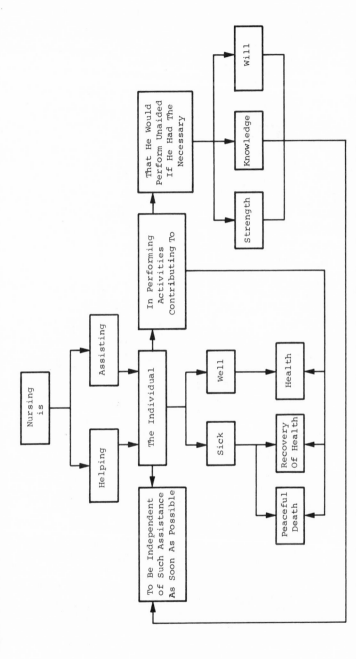

Figure 4-5 Dominant themes in Henderson's concept of nursing; formalization of patient agency theme and subsumption of health themes.

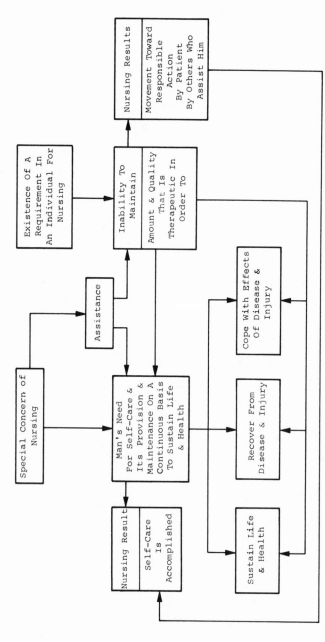

Figure 4-6 Dominant themes in Orem's concept of nursing; formalization of term *self-care*.

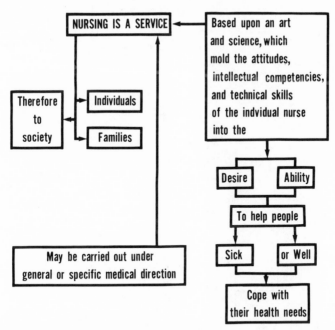

Figure 4-7 Dominant themes of the concept of nursing of Abdellah, Beland, Martin, and Matheney; focus on attributes of nurse as agent in relationship to patient agency.

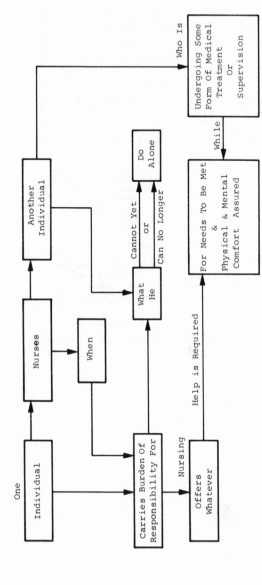

Figure 4-8 Dominant themes in Orlando's concept of nursing; formalization of nurse as responsible agent theme in relation to patient agency theme.

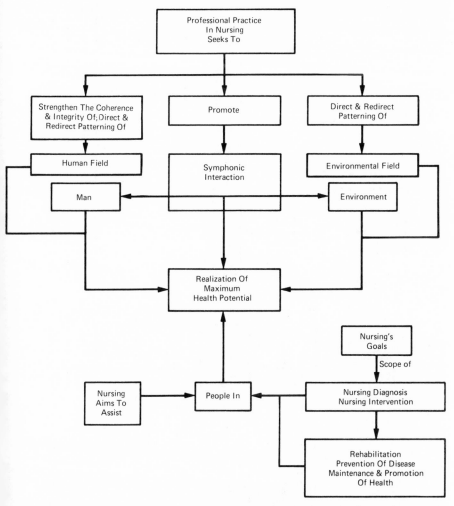

Figure 4-9   Dominant themes in Rogers' concepts of nursing focused on professional practice and nursing's aim and goals.

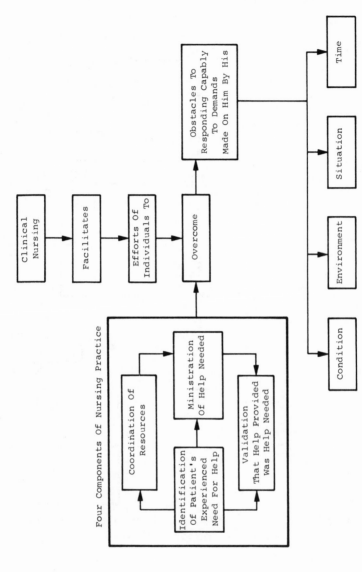

Figure 4-10 Dominant themes in Wiedenbach's concept of nursing; further development of patient agency theme.

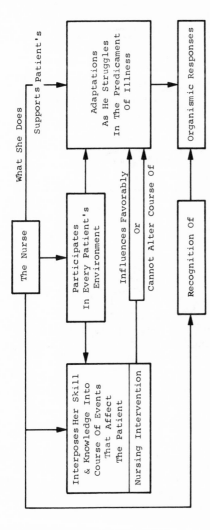

Figure 4-11 Dominant themes in Levine's concept of nursing focused on adaptations of ill patients.

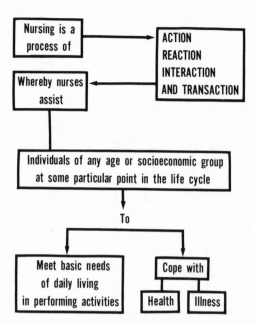

Figure 4-12 Dominant themes in King's concept of nursing; formalization of process elements and continuation of the basic needs and coping themes.

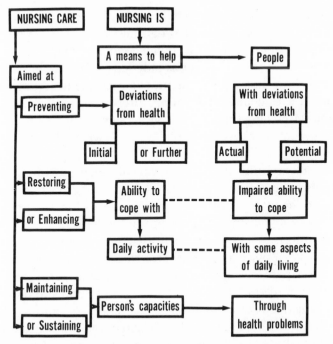

Figure 4-13 Dominant themes in Mitchell's concept of nursing; continued focus on patient agency, prevention, and coping themes.

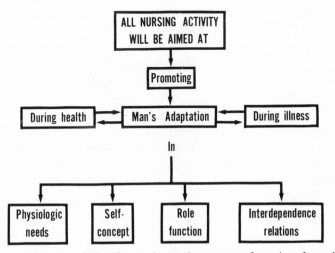

Figure 4-14 Dominant themes in Roy's concept of nursing; formalization of four modes of adaptation as focuses of nursing.

Recipients of nursing were identified as people (persons in general), for example, the Nightingale "us"; or as populations, persons of any age or socioeconomic group — the sick, the injured, the helpless; or as individuals who are in states of health or disease, dependent, experiencing needs, confronted with demands, adapting, interacting; or as agents. In some statements the recipient of nursing is referred to in a number of the above-described ways, as well as by the term *patient*.

Results of nursing and the forms of nursing action were expressed in a variety of ways. These are difficult to separate but, in the interests of exploring the range of ways of conceptualizing nursing, an attempt was made to sort them out.

Results of nursing were identified as including (1) states of persons expressed as readiness for the actions of "nature," or as related to health or disease; (2) states of persons expressed in relation to comfort and ease of mind and body; (3) adjustment of individuals to unalterable situations; (4) a peaceful death; (5) favorable or unfavorable adaptations of individuals; (6) health-care activities performed; (7) responsible actions of recipients of nursing in self-care; (8) freedom from assistance; (9) assumption of responsibility for care by members of the recipient's family or a non-nurse; (10) coherence and integrity of the "human field"; (11) "patterning of the human and environmental fields"; (12) judgments of the nurse; (13) meeting basic needs in performing activities of daily living; (14) ability to cope with daily living; or (15) modes of adaptation.

Characteristics of nursing as action were identified as including nursing conceptualized as (1) helping or assisting persons toward something or because of something; (2) activity that changes or in some way controls states of human beings or their environment (e.g., put, keep, facilitate, prevent, promote, conserve); (3) same as described in (2) but expressed in more specific terms (e.g., shelter, nourish); (4) assumption of or exercise of responsibility for another person; (5) "interposition of skills and knowledge," or manipulation of influencing factors; and (6) a "process of action, reaction, interaction, and transaction."

ADDITIONAL CONCEPTS

Three statements about the nature and goals of nursing that appeared in works that did not meet the criteria for inclusion in the sample are noted here. The nurses who expressed the ideas reported have been and are recognized for their contributions to theory development in nursing. The concepts of Hildegard Peplau, 1952, and Joyce Travelbee, 1966 and 1972, were contained in books written from a specialty perspective — interpersonal relations applicable to general nursing. Dorothy E. Johnson's conceptualizations were published in journal articles. Johnson has been credited by Roy and others for her influence on their work [27, pp. 35, 160].

Hildegard Peplau described nursing as a "human relationship" and formalized the dependency theme between an "individual who is sick, or in need of health services and a nurse especially educated to recognize and respond to the need for help" [29, pp. 5–6]. Peplau described a series of goal-directed steps in the process between the nurse and the recipients of nursing [29, p. 5]. "Effective nursing" according to Peplau means that "individuals and communities can be aided to use their capacities to bring about changes that influence living in desirable ways" [29, p. 8].

Joyce Travelbee's definition of nursing focuses upon the interpersonal process in which the professional nurse seeks to prevent or to help individuals to cope with "the experience of illness and suffering" and, if found necessary, help them "find meaning in the experience" [30, pp. 5–6; 31, p. 7].

In a 1961 journal article, *Dorothy Johnson's* conceptualization of nursing's responsibility was described in terms of assisting the patient "to maintain or reestablish equilibrium," a moving state, which occurs "throughout the health change process." Reduction of stress and tension and promotion of adaptation and stability are notions incorporated in Johnson's perspective [32, pp. 63–66].

CONCLUSIONS

The commonalities and differences in, as well as the structure of, the expressed general concepts of nursing afford some insights about the range of elements and relations expressed in general theories of nursing. Agreements are at a most general level: Nursing is action, a form of human service; it is concerned with man's functioning and states ensuing therefrom; it is a unique service in human society. The wide range of ways of conceptualizing nursing results (and this includes the contemporary period) would seem to indicate a need for discourse among scholars to consider each approach, to attach symbols to them, and to examine the implications of each for research methodologies.

Since the nature of nursing actions is related necessarily to results sought, it would be expected that examination of the results of nursing would force nurse scholars to attend to those phenomena of direct concern to nursing. This task would bring into consideration the elements and relations of expressed general concepts of nursing.

Identified elements and the relationships among them within the sample of statements about nursing, as well as the elements in statements by Peplau, Travelbee, and Johnson, do provide answers to the questions posed on the first page of this chapter. Further attention is needed to reveal their full meaning for nursing.

Scholarly endeavor directed toward classification and synthesis of the elements and relationships within the 17 expressions about nursing is suggested. The results of this endeavor would constitute a major contribution to the development of nursing as a discipline of knowledge.

The value of the 17 statements about nursing rests as much in their collective contribution to the affording of meaning to nursing as in their individual contributions.

REFERENCES

1. Maslow, A. *The Psychology of Science: A Reconnaisance.* New York: Harper & Row, 1966. Pp. 66–70.
2. Kaplan, A. *The Conduct of Inquiry.* San Francisco: Chandler, 1964. Pp. 46, 49.
3. Nightingale, F. *Notes on Nursing: What It Is and What It Is Not.* London: Harrison, 1859 and 1914 editions.

4. Nightingale, F. Sick Nursing and Health Nursing. In I. Hampton et al. (Eds.), *Nursing of the Sick, 1893*. New York: McGraw-Hill, 1949.

5. Shaw, C. S. W. *A Textbook of Nursing*. New York: Appleton, 1885 and 1902 (3rd) editions.

6. Harmer, B. *Text-Book of the Principles and Practice of Nursing*. New York: Macmillan, 1922.

7. Frederick, H. K., and Northam, E. *A Textbook of Nursing Practice* (2nd ed.). New York: Macmillan, 1938.

8. Harmer, B., revised by Henderson, V. *Textbook of the Principles and Practice of Nursing* (5th ed.). New York: Macmillan, 1955.

9. Henderson, V. *ICN Basic Principles of Nursing Care*. London: ICN (International Council of Nurses) House, 1960.

10. Henderson, V. *The Nature of Nursing*. New York: Macmillan, 1966.

11. Orem, D. E. *Guides for Developing Curricula for the Education of Practical Nurses*. Washington, D.C.: U.S. Government Printing Office, 1959.

12. Orem, D. E. *Nursing: Concepts of Practice*. New York: McGraw-Hill, 1971.

13. Nursing Development Conference Group. *Concept Formalization in Nursing: Process and Product*. Boston: Little, Brown, 1973.

14. Abdellah, F. G., Beland, I., Martin, A., and Matheney, R. *Patient-Centered Approaches to Nursing*. New York: Macmillan, 1960.

15. Abdellah, F. G., Beland, I., Martin, A., and Matheney, R. *New Directions in Patient Centered Nursing*. New York: Macmillan, 1973.

16. Orlando, I. J. *The Dynamic Nurse—Patient Relationship*. New York: Putnam's, 1961.

17. Orlando, I. J. *The Discipline and Teaching of Nursing Process: (An Evaluative Study)*. New York: Putnam's, 1972.

18. Rogers, M. *Educational Revolution in Nursing*. New York: Macmillan, 1961.

19. Rogers, M. *An Introduction to the Theoretical Basis of Nursing*. Philadelphia: Davis, 1970.

20. Wiedenbach, E. *Clinical Nursing: A Helping Art*. New York: Springer, 1964.

21. Wiedenbach, E. Nurses' wisdom in nursing theory. *Am. J. Nurs.* 70:1057—1062, 1970.

22. Levine, M. E. *Introduction to Clinical Nursing*. Philadelphia: Davis, 1969.

23. Levine, M. E. *Introduction to Clinical Nursing* (2nd ed.). Philadelphia: Davis, 1973.

24. King, I. E. *Toward a Theory for Nursing: General Concepts of Human Behavior*. New York: Wiley, 1971.

25. Mitchell, P. H. *Concepts Basic to Nursing*. New York: McGraw-Hill, 1973.

26. Mitchell, P. H. *Concepts Basic to Nursing.* New York: McGraw-Hill, 1977.
27. Riehl, J., and Roy, C. *Conceptual Models for Nursing Practice.* New York: Appleton-Century-Crofts, 1974.
28. Roy, C. *Introduction to Nursing: An Adaptation Model.* Englewood Cliffs, N.J.: Prentice-Hall, 1976.
29. Peplau, H. E. *Interpersonal Relations in Nursing: A Conceptual Frame of Reference for Psychodynamic Nursing.* New York: Putnam's, 1952.
30. Travelbee, J. *Interpersonal Aspects of Nursing.* Philadelphia: Davis, 1966.
31. Travelbee, J. *Interpersonal Aspects of Nursing* (2nd ed.). Philadelphia: Davis, 1971.
32. Johnson, D. E. The significance of nursing care. *Am. J. Nurs.* 61:63–66, 1961.

Formulations

5

A General Concept of Nursing System

PRELIMINARY WORK

The process of concept formalization engaged in by members of the NDCG enabled them in 1970 to enter the final stage of achievement of the expressed purpose of the NDCG's precursor, the Nursing Model Committee, a purpose formulated in 1965. In the early period of the work of the Committee,[1] members accepted the premise that a body of nursing knowledge is "at once a set of applied sciences and a practical science" [1]. The work accomplished up to 1970 by Group members was judged applicable to both forms of knowledge, but model development effort had contributed primarily to practical science considerations. This direction of effort resulted from the natural movement of the Group in its search of the order in nursing and from effort to work with Orem's general concept of nursing and, therefore, to consider nursing in its broadest dimensions.

This chapter describes the general concept of a nursing system developed by the NDCG, concentrating on identification and description of the elements of the system. "Practical science is one of action, behavior, conduct." It says "how we ought to behave and includes development of a method" [2]. A model for research in the art of nursing is a model for a "creative end product" and the end product is the test of the research. The creative end product comes into existence as a concept. The test to which the concept is put is twofold: (1) Can it be developed in the sector of reality? and (2) When developed does the result conform to the result conceptual-

---

[1] In the academic year, 1964—1965, Mary E. Redmond (deceased), at that time Dean of the School of Nursing, The Catholic University of America, arranged for W. A. Wallace, Ph.D. to conduct a series of faculty conferences on the nature and characteristics of the practical sciences and for E. F. O'Doherty, Ph.D., to work with the Nursing Model Committee and the Nursing Faculty on the logic of the nursing sciences.

ized? The problem of moving the theoretically conceived end product into the sphere of reality (the real world of nurses and patients) involves attention to the physics and mathematics of the problem(s) as well as to the natural science and technical science aspects of it.

The utility of a general concept of nursing in the sphere of practical science has been demonstrated through Group work.

THE CREATIVE END PRODUCT OF NURSING

In the work of identifying the dimensions of nursing as a practical science, the notion that *the creative end product of nursing is a nursing system* has emerged. The NDCG has worked with a concept of nursing system since 1968.[2] In November, 1970, a revised definition of nursing system was formulated following a three-day conference in August of the same year. This conference was concerned with summarization of the work efforts of the Group, including the articulation of subsidiary concepts and their relationships with the broad conceptual elements of Orem's general concept of nursing. This exercise produced models of the dominant themes of the general concept and sufficiently crystallized the formal relationships among the broad conceptual elements so that one member, a few weeks later, was able to formulate a definition of nursing system for consideration by the Group. The definition was accepted with the recognition that it expressed a general concept of nursing system and related it to a general concept of nursing and that these concepts were more theoretical and scientifically useful than the prior concepts used by the Group. The concerted and detailed group work with conceptual elements accomplished during the August conference was viewed as essential for the formalization of the revised concept of nursing system.

[2] A definition of *nursing system* was developed and revised by members of the Nursing Model Committee, The Catholic University of America, in 1968. The definition is presented in Chapter 6, p. 157.

A General Concept

The NDCG concept of nursing system as accepted in November, 1970, is presented with minor revisions in the statements that follow, with the suggestion that the creative end product of nursing is a nursing system. The form in which the conceptualizations are expressed is adapted from Ashby's description of the self-organizing system [3].

A *nursing system*, like other systems for the provision of personal services, is the product of a series of relations between persons who belong to different sets (classes), the set A and the set B. From a nursing perspective any member of the set A (legitimate patient) presents evidence descriptive of the complex subsets self-care agency and therapeutic self-care demand and the condition that in A demand exceeds agency due to health or health-related causes. Any member of the set B (legitimate nurse) presents evidence descriptive of the complex subset nursing agency which includes valuation of the legitimate relations between self as *nurse* and instances where, in A, certain values of the component phenomena of self-care agency and therapeutic self-care demand prevail.

B's perceptions of the conditionality of A's subset objective therapeutic self-care demand on the subset self-care agency establishes the conditionality of changes in the states of A's two subsets on the state of and changes in the state of B's subset nursing agency. The activation of the components of the subset nursing agency (change in state) by B to deliberately control or alter the state of one or both of A's subsets — therapeutic self-care demand and self-care agency — is nursing. The perceived relations among the parts of the three subsets (actual system) constitute the organization. The "mapping" of the behaviors in "mathematical or behavioral terms" provides a record of the system [4].

The concepts of nursing and nursing system expressed within the definition are recognized by the NDCG as exhibiting reliability and validity. The manner of symbolizing elements and the dynamics of the relations among them is viewed as a forward step in expressing the connotation of nursing when nursing is viewed as a practical science. It was anticipated that the concepts would be guides for more fruitful inquiry about (1) transformations of elements and transformations of their real-world referents and (2) transactions among the elements and transactions among their real-world referents.

The definition is based upon a number of presuppositions, including these assumptions:

1. Nursing is deliberate action, performed by individual persons on behalf of others, individually or in groups.
2. Deliberate actions performed by nurses on behalf of others are purposeful and organized; when actions are described in terms of their purposes and the relations among them the actions constitute a result-achieving process or a complex system of action.
3. Interpersonal relations between nurses and other persons (singly or in groups) who are recipients of nursing are essential if nursing is to occur.
4. Societies provide for the specialized position of the nurse and regulate the preparation and activities of persons in the position.
5. A general concept of nursing is essential for knowledge production in nursing since an adequate general concept of nursing makes explicit the proper object of nursing — that which is of direct concern to nurses (object of attention) and the way in which it is their concern.
6. Orem's concept of nursing at this stage in the development of nursing is an adequate concept.

These assumptions served as guides for formulating the concept of *what a nursing system is*, including the symbols utilized. The following statements may have value in clarifying the meaning of the expressed concept.

Referents and Symbols

The referents of Set A are persons in a society (now or in the future) who exhibit the condition specified, namely, that therapeutic self-care demand exceeds self-care agency due to some combination of health or health-related factors. The referents of Set A (legitimate patients of nurses) may be the object of attention of nurses either as individuals, as members of groups, or as segments of populations. It is suggested that, while particular forms of nursing practice may emphasize one or a combination of these views of persons, it may be essential for nurses to use all three views in a single nursing situation. For example, in community-health nursing a nurse may have as the focus of nursing practice the population of newborn infants in a community (a continuously changing population). Certain problems of providing nursing for a population of newborn infants are worked out at the population level. However, other problems of nursing related to the population must be handled at the level· of the individual infant and at the level of the family or other social unit of which the infant is a member. Each approach requires that the nurse use knowledge from a number of disciplines. The concomitant or sequential use of these approaches in nursing practice demands that the nurse have, be able to select from, and be able to apply relevant knowledge from the disciplines that focus on human beings as individuals, groups, and populations.

The term *set* is the *symbol* utilized to extend the object of nursing to all recipients of nursing (actual or potential). The term *legitimate* is utilized to designate that persons individually or as members of groups or populations possess that combination of characteristics or qualities that legitimates a relationship with a nurse, and which if initiated and established will afford them the social position of patient to a nurse.

The word *legitimate* as used here connotes *logical ideal (formal) admissibility* to a patient relationship with a nurse or nurses based on some conceptualization of what nursing is; *social admissibility* to such a relationship(s) based on cultural, including legal, norms; as well as actual *establishment of admissibility* by a nurse.

The symbols *self-care agency* and *therapeutic self-care demand* are utilized to stand for qualities or characteristics of, or judgments about, individuals, groups, or populations that are the direct concern of nursing and that are evaluated or made by nurses in their efforts to establish the existence of requirements for nursing. *Self-care agency* and *therapeutic self-care demand* are symbolized as subsets to connote that they are essential variables of the system. The real-world referents of each one are *a complement of qualities or phenomena or standards,* not a single referent. *Complex* is used as a modifier of subset to indicate this and also to indicate that the *entities within the subset* are related and that the *structuring of the relationships is not simple.*

In the definition of nursing system the *legitimacy of persons* (referents of Set B) holding, filling, or being qualified for the *position of nurse* in society is expressed in relation to persons having a set of *qualities or characteristics* symbolized by the term *nursing agency.* The statement makes explicit that the real-world referents of *nursing agency* in operation (activities or operations) include *valuations* of others to establish their legitimacy as *patients of nurses.* Nursing agency also includes operations through which nurses judge the adequacy of their own nursing agency as well as that of other nurses in specific situations. The valuing operations within the element nursing agency require that nurses utilize knowledge about nursing agency as an element of a nursing system, including its relations to the system elements self-care agency and therapeutic self-care demand.

Legitimate, subset, and *complex* are used in relation to nurses or nursing agency with the connotations described previously.

Explanatory Statements

The central focus of the definition of nursing system is nursing conceptualized as technology. The concept of nursing system contained in the definition sets forth elements and relations that are specifically the object of concern to nurses and not the object of concern to other health workers. The definition is not focused on nursing as an interpersonal system or on nursing's place in the larger social system. However, the essentiality of each of the foregoing is recognized and both are brought into relationships with the technologic nursing system. The technologic system is conceptualized as constituted in accord with the relations and the processes and transition probabilities between the two patient variables and between these variables and the nursing variable, nursing agency.

The general concept *system* was utilized as a vehicle, a means to (1) focus on elements and relations that are the direct concern of the nurse, separating these from a totality of elements and relations that are ascribed to individuals, groups, and populations [5] ; (2) place a *nursing system* within a network of interpersonal relations; and (3) separate persons involved into different sets according to the type and legitimacy of their positions and roles in the social order. The definition of nursing system expresses conceptualizations that indicate that nurses and recipients of nursing are involved in a hierarchy of interlocking systems — technologic, interpersonal, and social (Figure 5-1).

The decision to separate the technologic system and its elements from the interpersonal and social aspects of nursing practice had been made by the NDCG prior to the formulation of the definition presented in this chapter. (See Fig. 6-12).

A Triad of Systems   The concept of nursing system is expressed in terms of a deliberate relating of three elements: therapeutic self-care demand, self-care agency, and nursing agency. The elements are conceptualized as existing within interacting persons who have different qualities, occupy different statuses, and have different role sets. Various factors internal and external to the individuals in the system affect the system elements and their relations. This notion is illustrated in Figure 5-2.

Since the real-world referents of the elements of a nursing system (the technologic system) are attributed to human beings, a nursing system in this sense is dependent on the existence of an interpersonal system, a system of interaction that establishes linkages between persons who possess specified characteristics.

A nursing relationship between members of the Sets A and B is valid when these persons are legitimate incumbents of the positions *legitimate patient* and *legitimate nurse* as defined in the larger social system.

The initiation of a system of nurse—patient interaction between real persons in particular environmental settings (1) brings into reality certain stipulations and specifications for relations among persons of the society in which these persons

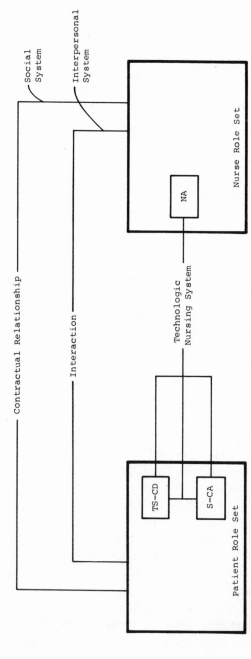

Figure 5-1 A hierarchy of interlocking systems. Key: TS–CD = therapeutic self-care demand, S–CA = self-care agency, NA = nursing agency.

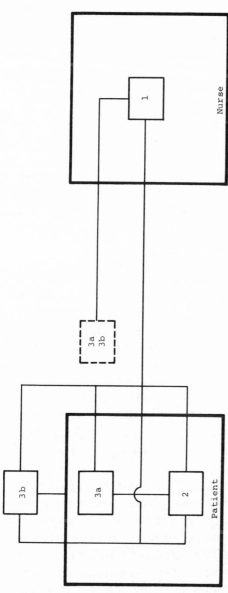

Figure 5-2 A nursing system — elements and relations. Key: 1, 2, 3 = system elements; 1 = nursing agency, 2 = self-care agency, 3a, 3b = therapeutic self-care demand, 3a = internally derived self-care requirements, 3b = externally derived self-care requirements.

113

live, and (2) sets in motion the application of rules of nursing practice as derived from the discipline, nursing. Thus, the interpersonal system serves an enabling function with respect to the technological and the social systems. There can be no nursing in a society without contact and association of individuals.

Interpersonal systems result from *contact and association* of individuals that make possible *interaction.* Interaction usually involves, and may require, deliberate communication using words or other symbols. In some instances, for example, when individuals know their roles in a social or technological system, the mere presence or state of one person is a stimulus for responsive action on the part of the other [6, 7].

The elements of interpersonal systems, contact and association of individuals and interaction, may be studied in terms of the variables of frequency, duration, and order [6, p. 14]. Interaction also can be studied in terms of one- or two-sidedness of interaction; extensity, intensity, and continuity of interaction; and its direction and organization [7, pp. 437–444].

Interpersonal systems generated by the interactions of nurses with recipients of nursing involve individuals in all their uniqueness as persons. Thus, the definition of nursing system, although technologically focused, specifies the approaches of *patient as person* and *nurse as person* as essential in nursing practice.

The interrelations among the three systems (Fig. 5-1) are matters of concern in nursing practice and in the development of nursing as a discipline. The NDCG suggests that the concept of nursing as a triad of systems has value (1) in determining the nature and dimensions of problems arising in nursing practice situations, and (2) in organizing knowledge now available for application in nursing practice. It would seem that, from the perspectives of theory development and research, attention should be given to each system individually, including points of articulation with other systems, as well as to the hierarchy as a total system.

A Triad of Elements   The three essential elements of a nursing system are described in terms of their characteristics and their functions in the system. Therapeutic self-care demand, because of its organizing role (serving to relate the other elements) in a nursing system, is described first.

Therapeutic self-care demand is a representational element in the sense that it is (at any point in time) (1) a summation of action to be taken, work to be done, (2) one standard against which the adequacy of self-care agency and nursing agency are assessed at any point in time, and (3) by virtue of the foregoing, a standard for deliberate change in the characteristics of self-care agency or nursing agency.

The qualitative and quantitative properties of therapeutic self-care demand serve as standards for the *nature* and the *frequency and duration of action* to be taken for the well-being of members of the Set A, legitimate patients. These properties are viewed in a nursing system in terms of their individual or combined effectiveness in maintaining A's biologic and rational life; bringing about or maintaining A's structural integrity or functioning within some designated range; or contributing to A's movement to a higher level of human functioning. Therapeutic self-care demand varies with factors internal to A and with factors in A's environment. The properties of the element can fluctuate over a wide range and the summation of demand for action may stabilize (for periods of long or short duration) at any point on the range over which its properties vary.

Therapeutic self-care demand is a conceptual product of legitimate patient or legitimate nurse or both derived from real-world elements. Once therapeutic self-care demand has been brought to the status of an element and maintained as an element in a nursing system through the judgments of A or B or both, its described representational functions are operative. For effectiveness of a nursing system, therapeutic self-care demand should be a joint product of the judgments of A and B except in instances where A cannot exercise agency.

Nursing agency is conceptualized as the prime regulatory mechanism for the nursing system (1) receiving *signals from* and *for* A as well as from B and from the environments of A and B, and interpreting the signals; and (2) on the basis of the meaning of the signals, regulating the flow of power that brings a nursing system into existence and maintains it in existence for some period of time. Signals are recognized through the operations of nursing agency. This involves comparing *some input* with *some standard* [8]. The meaning attached to the input from this comparison is a signal to B that nursing agency should or should not be further exercised with respect to members of the Set A. The exercise of nursing agency may be affected quantitatively (number of operations by time when required and time duration of each) and qualitatively (the nature of the operations, the degree of precision demanded, and the meaning of the operations for A in relation to change in, or degree of, control of self-care agency and therapeutic self-care demand).

Nursing agency in the concept nursing system is not only an essential element, an invariant, it also is the *principal part* of the system. It is through its exercise by legitimate nurses that nursing systems are conceptually created in relation to real-world phenomena internal or external to members of the Set A, brought into existence in the real world, and maintained and regulated for some period of time.

The exercise of nursing agency requires that members of the Set B who are able and willing to create nursing systems for others be in the physical presence of these others or, at least, be able to observe them and communicate with them through the use of information-transmitting media. Under the condition that the element self-care agency is wholly nonoperative or nondeveloped, it is a requirement of the system that B (or someone who will act under B's directions) be in the physical presence of A. Thus, two properties of self-care agency — the extent of its development and its operability at a particular time — specify the physical (spatial) relationship between A and B. When self-care agency is not operative or is undeveloped, *nursing agency* is the sole regulatory element in the system.

Self-care agency when developed and operative is viewed as a regulatory mechanism as described under nursing agency. Its operations may be directed to both of the other elements of the system — therapeutic self-care demand and nursing agency. Self-care agency is related to therapeutic self-care demand as a production mechanism (getting care accomplished) or as an estimating mechanism (determining what the demand is). Self-care agency as a production or estimating mechanism with respect to therapeutic self-care demand may be operative within or outside of a nursing system; in either situation the product of its exercise is a self-care system or some component thereof or a design for a self-care system.

The operations of self-care agency within a nursing system may be directed to transactions with nursing agency, including indications that transformations should occur in nursing agency. For example, A and B may deliberate their respective operations of agency with respect to therapeutic self-care demand; or A may represent to B facts that demand a change in nursing agency.

When both nursing agency and self-care agency are operative in a nursing system their relationship is mediated by therapeutic self-care demand as well as by the qualitative and quantitative properties of self-care agency [9].

When self-care agency is not operative the exercise of nursing agency must insure that effective substitutions for self-care agency are put into operation [9, p. 78].

In summary, it is the existence and operations of these elements, their properties, and the linkages among them that define the end product of nursing conceptualized by members of the NDCG as a nursing system.

DOMINANT THEMES OF THE CONCEPT NURSING SYSTEM

In summary, the three conceptualized elements within the concept nursing system are defined and further explained. The definitions suggest a beginning formalization of the con-

ceptual structure of each element and provide an orienting
framework for Chapter 6, which recounts the details of and
circumstances affecting the development of the elements of
the concept by the NDCG.

Self-Care Agency Defined

Self-care agency is the power of an individual to engage in the
estimative and production operations essential for self-care.
It is a complex, acquired quality that is described in terms of
abilities and limitations. Self-care refers to actions based on
culturally or scientifically derived practices freely performed
by individuals (or their agents), directed to themselves or to
conditions or objects in their environments in the interests
of their own life, health, or well-being [9, p. 13].

The characteristics of self-care agency described as abilities
and limitations are the results of certain factors, which include
growth and development state of the person; the state of human functioning; achieved purposive behavioral repertoire;
and the characteristics of the person's structured self-care
knowledge and developed self-care performance abilities.

The product of the exercise of self-care agency is the self-
care system or a design for it. The self-care behaviors from
which the system emerges at a point in time are a portion of
the behavioral repertoire, which is self-care agency. The self-
care system is a segment of the person's system of daily living.
If the focus of attention is the system of daily living, the
self-care system may then be viewed as a subsystem of the
larger system.

The person having self-care agency exists in an environment
that has an effect on the development of, the exercise of,
and the demand on self-care agency. The demand on self-
care agency as perceived by the person and as reflected through
knowledge, experience, and image of oneself as self-care agent
activates components of the existent behavioral repertoire
which constitutes self-care agency.[3]

[3]Some results of continuing efforts to formalize the structure of self-care agency
are presented in Chapters 7 and 8.

Therapeutic Self-Care Demand Defined

Therapeutic self-care demand is a complex of objectively established requirements for action (including qualitative, quantitative and time specifications) that would assist a person with the maintenance of present states of health or well-being or with movement toward estimated desirable states. The demand when formulated is essentially a design for actions to be taken: The design makes explicit the reasons for the actions, the nature of the actions, the relationships among sets of actions, and the expected results of action that are stipulated as required by, or desirable for, a person. The action requirements that are the constitutive parts of therapeutic self-care demand are described as *universal self-care requirements* or *health-deviation self-care requirements* [9, pp. 20–30]. Specifications for meeting requirements may include sets of actions that are designed to link a person's self-care system to a larger health-care system.

Therapeutic self-care demand is formulated by a process of associating practices that have a demonstrated range of instrumental effectiveness or are hypothesized as effective with data constituting evidence of a need to (1) change or (2) maintain intrahuman or extrahuman factors at some value level.

An adequate formulation of therapeutic self-care demand includes sets of actions related to (1) the individual's becoming, being, or remaining self-actuating in an external environment; (2) maintaining or restoring or controlling effectiveness of functioning within a range of values at levels ranging from the molecular to the uniquely human; and (3) prevention or control of structural changes due to forces internal or external to the person.

The experiencing of the therapeutic self-care demand by a person activates self-care agency. Action of the person directed to meet in part, or to refrain from meeting, the therapeutic self-care demand forms the self-care system. The qualitative and quantitative adequacy of a self-care system is judged in terms of its total or partial instrumental effectiveness in meeting the therapeutic self-care demand.

Nursing Agency Defined

Nursing agency is a complex set of qualities of a person acquired through specialized study and experiences in real-world nursing situations. This set of qualities enables a person to assist others (1) in the immediate exercise of self-care agency, in its initial or continuing development, or in making transformations in it, but always in relation to the person's usual pattern of self-care or the objectively established therapeutic self-care demand; (2) by determining the constitutive parts of therapeutic self-care demand and the essential relations among the parts, and by keeping therapeutic self-care demand adjusted to changes in the person or the environment (this includes the availability of valid and reliable technologies); (3) by evaluating the characteristics of the individual's self-care system(s) with respect to adequacy as related to an objectively established therapeutic self-care demand; (4) by designing and assisting with the institution and management of self-care systems that relate various abilities within self-care agency to parts, or to the totality, of self-care demand; and (5) by designing and providing systems of assistance that substitute for the total or partial absence of self-care agency or compensate for specific inadequacies of the constitutive parts of self-care agency.

The general characteristics of nursing agency are described as nursing abilities and limitations as related to the aforementioned types of assistance adjusted to conditions prevailing in some types of nursing situations. The characteristics of nursing agency at a specific time are the result of certain enabling and limiting factors related to a nurse's age and maturity, degree of development and perfection of the nursing art, structured nursing knowledge, state of health, and the environmental conditions under which the nurse exercises nursing agency.

The nursing behaviors that a nurse activates in a particular nursing situation at a particular time are only a portion of the total behavioral repertoire of nursing agency. Nursing agency is activated initially by stimuli and signals relevant to establishing the characteristics of, and making judgments about, constitutive parts of *therapeutic self-care demand and self-care agency.* Subsequent activation of nursing agency results from judgments about: (1) the presence, the causes, and the dimensions of a *self-care deficit;* (2) the possibility or feasibility of *effecting transformations in self-care agency* as related to therapeutic self-care demand; and (3) effective methods to meet specific action requirements within therapeutic self-care demand now, in the immediate future, and in the more distant future.

These three sets of judgments establish the conditionality of changes in self-care agency and therapeutic self-care demand on the exercise of nursing agency. When the conditionalities are established, further exercise of nursing agency will be directed toward the achievement of some combination of results expressed in relation to therapeutic self-care demand and self-care agency. Results that accrue over time include the following:

1. Self-care agency is or is becoming proportionate to estimating and meeting therapeutic self-care demand.
2. Self-care agency is exercised in relation to therapeutic self-care demand, and this exercise produces a self-care system that exhibits effectiveness in meeting constitutive parts, or the totality, of the demand.
3. Therapeutic self-care demand at any point in time (a) describes factors in the patient or the environment that (for the sake of the patient's life, health, or well-being) must be held steady within a range of values or brought within and held within such a range, and (b) has a known degree of instrumental effectiveness derived from the choice of technologies and specific techniques for use in changing, or in some way controlling, patient or environmental factors.
4. Therapeutic self-care demand is met over time.

Nursing agency has been described as the power of one individual to provide for other individuals with health-related self-care deficits material and energy inputs essential for the self-maintenance and the health and well-being of these others. Nursing agency is exercised in the form of a dynamic system of human actions. The end product of the exercise of nursing agency is this dynamic system of action (a nursing system), which must be brought into existence, maintained in existence, and managed to accomplish for legitimate patients some or all of the four results described previously.

FOUNDATIONAL CONCEPTS
At the level of greatest generality there are five concepts that underlie the subject matter of nursing and provide subsuming or organizing framework for foundational material in cognitive structure [10]. These concepts are man, action, process, organization, and system. Each concept is broad and can be viewed by scholars or disciplines in a variety of ways. It is essential, therefore, that the Group make each foundational concept explicit in a formalized statement indicating how each concept articulates most accurately with the general concept of nursing system.

Man
The term *man* is used in the sense of *human beings collectively*. The term *individual* or *individual human being* rather than the term man is used to refer to a human being as *one of a species* or as a *member of a population*. Closely associated with the terms man and individual is the term person. *Person* is used to refer to individual human beings when conceptualized in the *fullness of their being human*. The reference then is to their *individuality* expressed as a unity of being and becoming; of knowing, feeling, and imagining; of reflecting and judging; of valuing and willing; and to their possession of self by self [11, 12, 13]. The person is revealed to others through developed and unique modes of relating to the environment. Allport refers to this as "personality" [13, pp. 61, 89–92].

Whenever the terms *individual human being* and *person* are used the referent is a human individual, an existent unity, a dynamic being in a continuing process of development. Unity therefore is accepted as integral to man as a human being and not as a special way of viewing man. The special characteristics of the unitary nature of man can be explored metaphysically, as was done by Lonergan who, in using and explaining the genetic or developmental method, viewed human organic, psychic, and intellectual development as interlocking levels of integrations [12, pp. 469–479]. Nurses deal with themselves and others in the concreteness of their individuality. Knowledge of the persuasive (heuristic) arguments and categories of metaphysicians can lead nurses to explore themselves and others as "beings in process" [12, pp. 625–626].

The NDCG accepts that the proper object of a discipline, including the practice disciplines, specifies that which members of the particular discipline should apprehend and know in the world of man. The NDCG further accepts that the proper object of nursing, as a practice discipline, is or should be expressed (or is implicit) in developed and valid general concepts of nursing. The NDCG takes the position that the view or views of man that are nursing-specific are expressed or are implicit in formulated general theories or concepts of nursing. In light of the NDCG's expressed concept of nursing system and assuming interlocking levels of lower to higher integrations in man as a "being in process," for its purposes the NDCG takes a four-dimensional view of man. For nursing purposes man is viewed variously as *agent, symbolizer, organism,* and as *object* (subject to physical forces). The following definition of man incorporates the four dimensions.

Definition   Man is a psychophysiologic organism with rational powers. As a biological organism man exists, and responds both as organism and object, in an environment with physical and biological components. As a rationally functioning being, man symbolizes and formulates purposes about, and acts on, self, others, and the environment.

Action
Action theory (including concepts of action) has been of value in the formalization of nursing concepts and in sorting out empirical data.

Definition Action is behavior of a person that is deliberate and intended to affect something to which it is directed, moving it to a condition that differs from its condition prior to being acted upon [14]. Action is particular to the person who endeavors to change or prevent change or preserve the state of something (self, other persons, objects, or environmental conditions).

Action always involves time. It involves knowledge to provide structure, feeling or motivation to provide energy, and movement of the person in relation to a former situation; all are bound together in a unity that is action [14, pp. 86, 128; 15].

Process

Process is the subsuming concept most relevant to the technologies that are the products of the practical sciences in nursing. Technology as process is the means of converting order from what would otherwise be random results [16].

Definition ". . . an act is always a process in time" [17]. Process is a continuous and regular action or succession of actions taking place or carried on in a definite manner [18]. Process involves the coordination of the activities of the actor. The object or goal that the actor intends to bring about defines the manner of acting (i.e., the direction and nature of the actions) and the simultaneous or sequential performance of actions so that they have facilitating or impeding relations one to the other [19]. Achievement of the goal sets the limit on the time dimension of the process.

Organization

Since a general concept of organization subsumes concepts of order and relations among real or conceptualized parts of some whole, it is a useful conceptual tool in analysis and synthesis and in concept formalization. A general concept of organization and a concept of a specific form of organization are presented. Both concepts have utility in nursing.

Definition   Organization is an arrangement of parts in relation one to the other so that the parts work as a unit. The
concept of organization reflected in the NDCG concept of
nursing system — that relations between two entities A and
B are conditional on C's value or state — is an acceptance of
that of Ashby [3].

Organization also is defined as "a system of consciously
coordinated activities or forces of two or more persons" [20].
This definition of organization places primary emphasis on
the linkages in the actions of two or more persons. The change
in the other that would be intended in these actions is from
individual action to cooperative action. Organizations can be
viewed from a structural perspective — the summary but
stationary definition of positions and descriptions of responsibilities and of the linkages through which coordinated action
is accomplished [20, p. 119]. The essence of the organization
exists in the coordinated action, which has as its purpose the
overcoming of limitations restricting what individuals can do
alone [20, p. 23].

System

The Group first utilized a general concept of system and
more recently a concept of a specific type of system.

Definition   A system is "sets of objects together with relationships between the objects and between their attributes"
[21]. The objects constituting the system behave together
as a whole; changes in any part affect the whole [3, pp. 108–
118].

A variety of types of systems can be viewed within this
general framework. The type of system most accurately suited
to practical science purposes in nursing is the self-organizing
system.

Self-organizing systems are those that exist only when and
for the duration that there are self-connecting links between
the behavior or state of independent parts or subjects, the
connection occurring at some point of conditionality between
them [3, pp. 108–118].

REFERENCES

1. O'Doherty, E. F.   Notes from the May 13, 1965, Meeting of the Nursing Model Committee, Faculty of Nursing, The Catholic University of America, Washington, D.C.
2. O'Doherty, E. F.   Notes from the May 20, 1965, Meeting of the Nursing Model Committee, Faculty of Nursing, The Catholic University of America, Washington, D.C.
3. Ashby, W. R.   Principles of the Self-Organizing System. In W. E. Buckley (Ed.), *Modern Systems Research for the Behavioral Scientist.* Chicago: Aldine, 1968. P. 108.
4. Nursing Development Conference Group.   Minutes of the Meeting of Nov. 13—14, 1970 (typewritten). P. 4. (Revised Aug., 1971.)
5. Sagasti, F.   A Conceptual and Taxonomic Framework for the Analysis of Adaptive Behavior. In L. von Bertalanffy and A. Rapoport (Eds.), *General Systems, XV.* Washington, D.C.: Society for General Systems Research, 1970. P. 151.
6. Homans, G.   Elements of Behavior. In D. W. Minar and S. Greer (Eds.), *The Concept of Community.* Chicago: Aldine, 1969. Pp. 13—15.
7. Sorokin, P.   *Social and Cultural Dynamics.* Boston: Extending Horizons Books, Porter Sargent, 1957. Pp. 438—444.
8. Vickers, G.   A Classification of Systems. In L. von Bertalanffy and A. Rapoport (Eds.), *General Systems, XV.* Washington, D.C.: Society for General Systems Research, 1970. P. 3.
9. Orem, D. E.   *Nursing: Concepts of Practice.* New York: McGraw-Hill, 1971. Pp. 79—80.
10. Ausubel, D. P.   Some Psychological Aspects of the Structure of Knowledge. In *Education and the Structure of Knowledge.* Chicago: Rand McNally, 1964. Pp. 221—249.
11. Maritain, J.   *The Degrees of Knowledge.* New York: Scribner's, 1959. P. 231.
12. Lonergan, B. J. F.   *Insight.* New York: Philosophical Library, 1957. Pp. 266—267.
13. Allport, G. W.   *Becoming.* New Haven: Yale University Press, 1955. Pp. 41—56.
14. Macmurray, J.   *Self as Agent.* London: Faber & Faber, 1966. Pp. 55, 101.
15. Piaget, J.   *Psychology of Intelligence.* Totowa, N.J.: Littlefield, Adams, 1969. P. 4.
16. Young, T. R.   Social Stratification and Modern Systems Theory. In L. von Bertalanffy and A. Rapoport (Eds.), *General Systems, XIV.* Washington, D.C.: Society for General Systems Research, 1969. Pp. 113—117.

17. Parsons, T. *The Structure of Social Action.* New York: Macmillan Free Press Paperback, 1968. Vol. 1, p. 45.
18. *The Oxford Universal Dictionary.* New York: Oxford University Press, 1955. P. 1590.
19. Kotarbinski, T. *Praxiology* (translated by O. Wojtasiewicz). New York: Pergamon, 1965. P. 47.
20. Barnard, C. *The Functions of the Executive.* Cambridge: Harvard University Press, 1966. P. 73.
21. Hall, A. D., and Fagan, R. E. Definition of System. In L. von Bertalanffy and A. Rapoport (Eds.), *General Systems,* I. Ann Arbor: Society for General Systems Research, 1956. P. 18.

6

Dynamics of Concept Development

The NDCG's definition of nursing system emerged from the work of the Group. This work included consideration and application of generalizations from works concerned with general systems theory, organizational theory, and action theory and those concerned with man as unified being affected by, or affecting, elements within the larger whole of which man is a part.

The 1970 general concept of nursing system is considered within the Group as a forward movement in the development of "manageable models" or "simplified approximations" of the multiplicity of actions, events, or results which together constitute the provision of nursing to members of a society. The conceptualizations of legitimate patient, legitimate nurse, and the elements self-care agency, therapeutic self-care demand, and nursing agency are in the nature of static concepts, abstractions, which are "dominant enough" to unite secondary concepts that form the substantive structure of each dominant theme.

This chapter presents descriptions of the process of development of the dominant themes incorporated within the NDCG's general concept of nursing system. Work from 1965 to 1971 directed toward the development of dominant themes represents the members' attempts to construct a conceptual framework and to validate the conceptual framework by analyses of descriptions of nursing situations. The utilization of the concept as a structuring framework for reality situations in nursing represents a research effort utilizing the method of developing a creative end product. Both processes contribute evidence to the adequacy of the general concept of nursing system presented in Chapter 5.

This chapter also presents the work of the Group related to the identification of factors that condition the values of the nursing system variables with a focus on the patient variables, self-care agency, and therapeutic self-care demand.

Group deliberations about relations of the views of man specific to nursing as a practice discipline to the patient variables of nursing systems and to factors that condition the values of the variables are summarized.

DOMINANT THEMES

The development of the "dominant themes" or the "high spots" of a general concept of nursing is essential in establishing the reliability and validity of the concept. Once developed, the secondary concepts within the dominant themes serve to establish a framework for integrating segments of theory from other disciplines and to provide some direction to the selection of useful research methodologies for study of reality situations. The essence of the initial work of dominant theme development is the formalization of static concepts that serve to give a nursing structure to a range of real-world phenomena involved in the provision of nursing in a society. Dominant theme development involves the acceptance and systematic use in real nursing situations of elements and relations specified within a general concept of nursing.

Development enters a dynamic and productive stage when the substantive structure of the elements emerges, with the result that the relationships become more specifically described in terms of identified and conceptualized qualitative or quantitative characteristics of the elements. This work also is fruitful in the isolation of research methodologies of nursing and, thus, in the development of the syntactical structure of nursing.

The static concepts of self-care agency, therapeutic self-care demand, and nursing agency, which emerged in a 1970 session of the NDCG, will be presented and explored from a historical and developmental perspective. This will incorporate the work of the Group when it met as the Nursing Model Committee (April, 1965, to May, 1968), a subcommittee of the Graduate Curriculum Committee of the School of Nursing, The Catholic University of America, and as the Nursing Development Conference Group (September, 1968), a formal but voluntary study group that exists outside the structure of any larger organization.

Self-Care Agency

In the Group's concept of nursing system, *self-care agency* is one of two patient characteristics whose value conditions the nursing agency, which is made operative to achieve health care for individuals or groups in reality situations. In the development of Group thinking about this quality, the more concrete element, *self-care,* occupied an important basic position in work sessions. Self-care was the primary focus of discussion in the early sessions of the Group. Exploration centered on the nature and amount of responsibility for care of self that patients might maintain while under the care of a nurse. The vehicle for discussion was *individual cases* or *categories of patients* (the unconscious patient, the conscious but paralyzed patient, the child) or general questions such as the *relation between habit and voluntary action.* From the content of these discussions, tentative generalizations were derived.

The initial formal meeting of the first Nursing Model Committee was held in April, 1965; at that time the committee reviewed and revised four sets of *propositions about self-care* which had been formulated by one of its members, Dorothea Orem, for her own writings. Group effort was directed toward devising methods to check the validity of the generalizations. Work took place predominantly at the monthly committee meetings during the period of two academic years. Patient situations were analyzed in Group sessions to determine whether the concept (self-care) was useful in handling data from reality situations. During review of a film, *The Special Universe of Walter Krolic,*[1] a section of the members attempted to identify *evidences of self-care conduct* in the behaviors

---

[1] The Group recognized that the film depicted a fictional rather than a real patient. It was assumed that the film script reflected the reality of nursing situations of this type.

of the patient portrayed in the film. From the viewpoint of exploratory analysis, the use of a film had several advantages. It maintained members in face-to-face contact so that exchange of ideas could occur. It exposed them to the same portrayed events. Sequences of the film could be rerun for comparative examination without affecting the original stimulus. This method was useful in allowing members to explore *whether they were utilizing the terms of the element as a consistent symbolization of the same conceptual and reality phenomena* (as portrayed in the film).

Following each of these activities, the sets of propositions about self-care were revised. The terminal point for this work was contained in a 1967 report in which a series of accepted and partially validated statements about self-care were offered for faculty consideration in a Committee report. The statements were developed in the form of a set of premises and three sets of propositions. The premises, which are presented below, are a revised version of the first set of the 1965 propositions; the major revision made explicit the relationship between self-care and society.

SOME PREMISES ABOUT SELF-CARE

1. Self-care is conduct. It is ego-processed. It is a learned activity, learned through interpersonal relations and communications.
2. Each adult person has the right and responsibility to care for himself to maintain his rational life and health; he may have such responsibilities for other persons.
   a. Infant and child care, care of the aged, and care of the adolescent include the giving, assisting with, or supervising the self-care of another.
   b. Social assistance will be needed by an adult person whenever the person is unable to obtain needed resources and maintain conditions necessary for the preservation of life and promotion of health for himself or for his dependents; such assistance may be needed for the accomplishment or the supervision of self-care [1].

The three sets of propositions in the 1967 report incorporate Sets 2 to 4 of the 1965 propositions. Changes appear in the form of revisions and expansions, both of which give greater recognition to the effect of psychologic and social factors on self-care. The expanded integration of these two disciplines, psychology and sociology, is in part the result of interim contact with a consultant (Eamonn F. O'Doherty, Ph.D., Chairman, Department of Psychology, University College, Dublin) who had worked with the faculty several years in succession. The propositions appeared as follows:

SOME PROPOSITIONS ABOUT SELF-CARE

Set One — Conditioning Factors

1. Self-care conduct is affected by self-concept and by the level of maturity of the individual.
2. Self-care conduct is affected by culturally derived goals and practices.
3. Self-care conduct is affected by the scientifically derived health knowledge possessed by a person.
4. Self-care conduct is affected by placement in the family constellation.
5. Self-care conduct is affected by membership in social groups exclusive of the family, for example, friendship and work groups.
6. Adults may or may not choose to engage themselves in specific self-care actions.
7. Lack of scientifically derived knowledge about self-care, disorders of health and malfunctioning, lack of self-care skills, and inadequate habits of self-care limit what a person can do with respect to his own self-care or in assisting another person in such matters.

Set Two — Self-Care in Health and Disease

1. Self-care contributes to and is necessary for a person's integrity as a psychophysiologic organism with a rational life.
2. Each person must perform or have performed for him each day a minimum of activities directed to, or performed for the sake of, himself in order to continue his existence as an organism with a rational life. If health is to be maintained and improved, he must perform additional activities. In the event of disease, injury, or mental or physical malfunctioning he must perform other activities to sustain life or improve health.
3. Self-care directed to the maintenance and promotion of health requires a scientifically derived fund of knowledge about self-care goals and practices as well as related skills and habits.
4. Disease, injury, and mental or physical malfunctioning may limit what a person can do for himself, since such states may limit his ability to reason, to make decisions, and to engage in activity to accomplish self-care goals. Disease, injury, and malfunctionings may involve structural changes as well as functional changes, which may necessitate the use of specialized self-care measures, some of which may be medically prescribed.

Set Three — Behavioral and Resource Demands of Self-Care

1. Self-care requires general knowledge of self-care goals and practices as well as specific knowledge about self, including health state, and about the physical and social environment. It also requires internalization of insights and sanctions and motivation. Acquiring specific knowledge involves making observations and judgments and leads to understanding of present self-care requirements as well as the self-care deficit; it may require contact and interactions with workers in the health services.

2. Self-care includes seeking and participating in medical care prescribed by the physician in the event of deviations or departures from health, and periodic scientific evaluations of health states.

3. Self-care requires internally oriented activities directed to the control of behavior; self-care also requires externally oriented behavior directed to the control of the environment, to establishing contact and communication with others, and to the securing and utilization of resources.

4. Self-care requires the use of resources that may include living in a healthful or a therapeutic physical and social environment; consumption of water, food, and drugs; application of physical agents and drugs to external surfaces and to those internal surfaces that communicate with the exterior; introduction of drugs into the body tissues to supply substances that the body is not producing; use of artificial devices to control the position of the body or its parts, or to aid in movement; use of prosthetic devices to facilitate functioning [1, pp. 3–4].

The 1967 statement represents the culmination of the original Group's work on the *formalization of the concept of self-care*. The fact that the term *self-care conduct* was the prevalent symbol reflects the essence of the concept: *self-care is behavior; it exists in reality situations.*

The term *agency* has been attached to the *concept of self-care* since the inception of the NDCG. The term has been consistently used since a meeting (August, 1969) in which the Group members examined and attempted to illustrate their *view of man* and of the *relationship of agency factors to this view.* This addition made explicit the position of the Group within *action theory.* It was also in keeping with the *developing systems orientation* in the Group's work [2].

During the NDCG's existence, the most extensive effort in relation to the concept of self-care agency has been toward the conceptual and empirical exploration of the dimensions of, and associations within, the concept. Early in the history of the Group (May, 1965), members accepted the recommendation of a consultant (O'Doherty) that the *concept of research not be limited to that of experimental sciences.* It was accepted that in the beginning stages of discipline development, *natural history method* and the *hypothetical deductive method* are of value in the identification of elements within the concepts and of linkages between the elements.

A 1956 article by Ashby [3] lent validity to the approach. In the article he indicated that the strategy of varying one factor is of use only when the system is fairly simple. Although in terms of persons, a nurse and a patient, the nursing system may appear to be simple, it was the position of the Group that the major focus of the system was not the persons themselves but a complexity of complementary elements that had to be coordinated between and within them. Thus it seemed reasonable to accept Ashby's emphasis that search be directed in a manner that could deal with relations and the process and transition probabilities, which establish the flexible structure.

One of the initial efforts in the area of research in relation to self-care was undertaken independently of committee work but under the direction of one of its members. Louise Hartnett (who joined the Group in October, 1968) completed a study that utilized the Group's concept of nursing to organize knowledge concerning the maintenance of normal body temperature around the concepts of self-care agency and therapeutic self-care demands and deficits [4]. Using the hypothetical deductive method, a series of theoretical models were developed. Literature in the fields of physiology, psychology, and human behavior was analyzed to develop a conceptualization of voluntary human action involving motor activity. Two complementary models were developed to make explicit what is involved physiologically and psychologically in self-care agency [4, pp. 69, 87] (see Figs. 6-1 through 6-5).

Literature in the fields of physiology and bioclimatology was identified and analyzed to extract items descriptive of

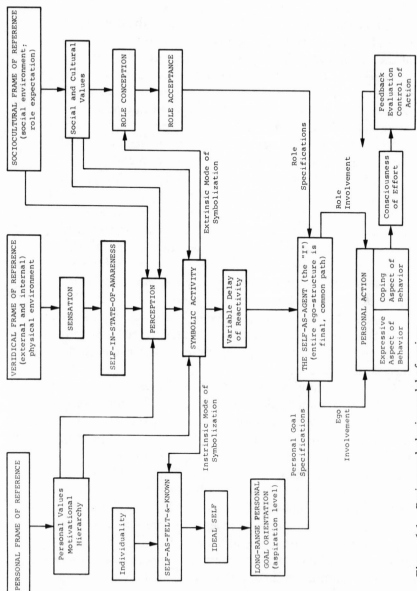

Figure 6-1 Basic psychologic model of action.

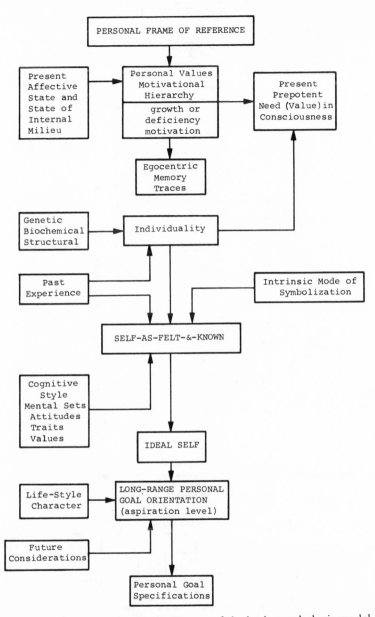

Figure 6-2   Personal frame of reference of the basic psychologic model of action.

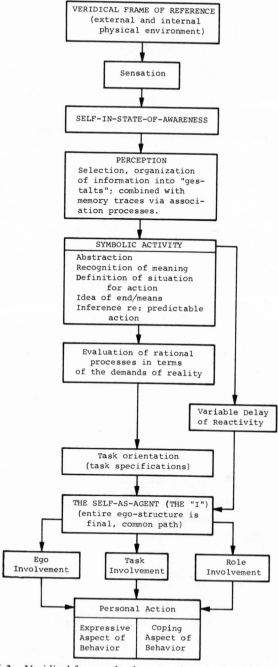

Figure 6-3 Veridical frame of reference of the basic psychologic model of action.

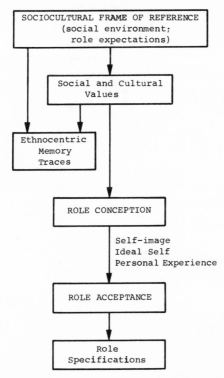

Figure 6-4   Sociocultural frame of reference of the basic psychologic model of action.

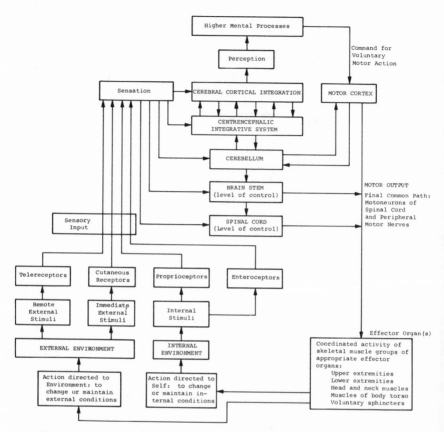

Figure 6-5 Physiologic model of action.

man's physiologic regulative and adaptive mechanisms in various thermal environments and his cultural and technologic efforts to supplement his physiologic adaptation. The literature documented the maintenance of normal body temperature as an aspect of self-care, deliberate, purposive human action to maintain life and health. Through a process of documentary analysis of this literature, partial models concerning the physiologic and psychologic aspects of maintaining normal body temperature were developed and studied in relation to the models descriptive of aspects of self-care agency.

In the last phase of the study, models setting forth the essential elements and relationships that might guide the determination of nursing requirements in the area of maintaining normal body temperature were developed — a model of the major forms of self-care valid for the maintenance of normal body temperature and a guide to nursing assessment in the area of maintaining normal body temperature under various external thermal conditions.

The study also provided a basis for the development and validation of scientifically based nursing action systems relative to maintaining normal body temperature.

The model setting forth some of the dimensions of self-care agency, which is one of a series of models developed in the study, is presented here as Figure 6-6 [4, p. 181].

Review of the Hartnett study by the NDCG members was a transitional phase in the Group work. Following its review and discussion, focus of effort shifted from conceptualization about self-care to examination of ways to explore the reality through *development of techniques for collection and analysis of data about self-care agency.* Patient data were collected over time and members began or continued to record their own self-care practices, collecting these data over time. Examination of some of the available case material in Group sessions has led to the *evolution of models for sorting data,* and of *models describing processes involved in self-care agency.* The remainder of the material was held for more careful and consistent analysis.

Figure 6-7 depicts the framework of certain factors identified as relevant to assess the agency status of persons having ongoing disease processes. The framework provided the Group with a mechanism for sorting patient data and for identifying some relationships between conceptualized elements. Figure 6-8 depicts the utilization of the model in the handling of data about one patient [5].

Figure 6-9 establishes a framework for identifying and organizing knowledge on which health action and deliberate action are based [6]. Knowledge of the factors and processes involved in self-care action exists, at least in part, in the doer of the action, whether this be the patient or the nurse. Organization of the knowledge of action components into ranges and dimensions is a function of a discipline. When applied to

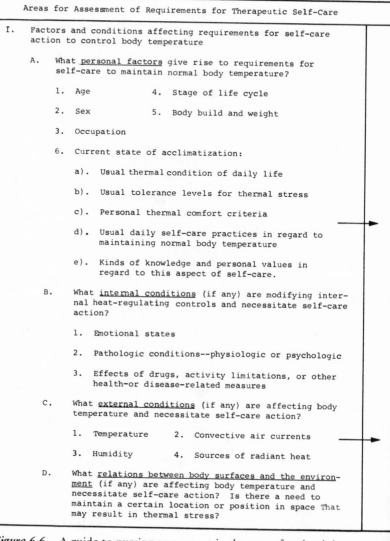

Areas for Assessment of Requirements for Therapeutic Self-Care

I. Factors and conditions affecting requirements for self-care action to control body temperature

   A. What <u>personal factors</u> give rise to requirements for self-care to maintain normal body temperature?

      1. Age   4. Stage of life cycle

      2. Sex   5. Body build and weight

      3. Occupation

      6. Current state of acclimatization:

         a). Usual thermal condition of daily life

         b). Usual tolerance levels for thermal stress

         c). Personal thermal comfort criteria

         d). Usual daily self-care practices in regard to maintaining normal body temperature

         e). Kinds of knowledge and personal values in regard to this aspect of self-care.

   B. What <u>internal conditions</u> (if any) are modifying internal heat-regulating controls and necessitate self-care action?

      1. Emotional states

      2. Pathologic conditions--physiologic or psychologic

      3. Effects of drugs, activity limitations, or other health-or disease-related measures

   C. What <u>external conditions</u> (if any) are affecting body temperature and necessitate self-care action?

      1. Temperature   2. Convective air currents

      3. Humidity   4. Sources of radiant heat

   D. What <u>relations between body surfaces and the environment</u> (if any) are affecting body temperature and necessitate self-care action? Is there a need to maintain a certain location or position in space That may result in thermal stress?

Figure 6-6 A guide to nursing assessment in the area of maintaining normal body temperature.

self-care, the knowledge is accepted as uniquely nursing.

Figures 6-7 and 6-8 are examples of the *models abstracted from the case material about self-care* that had been collected on patients or on members of the Group. The nature of the

irements For .f-Care .ction to intain ormal Body perature →

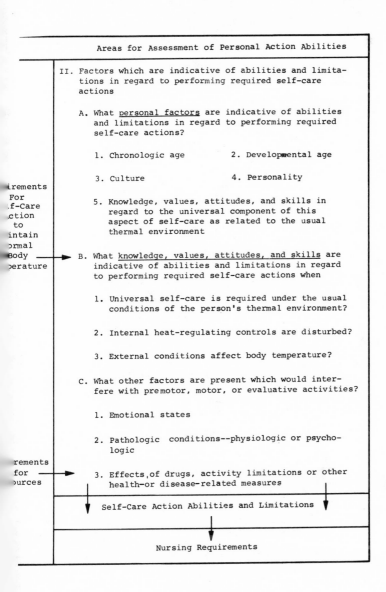

Areas for Assessment of Personal Action Abilities

II. Factors which are indicative of abilities and limitations in regard to performing required self-care actions

A. What <u>personal factors</u> are indicative of abilities and limitations in regard to performing required self-care actions?

1. Chronologic age
2. Developmental age
3. Culture
4. Personality
5. Knowledge, values, attitudes, and skills in regard to the universal component of this aspect of self-care as related to the usual thermal environment

B. What <u>knowledge, values, attitudes, and skills</u> are indicative of abilities and limitations in regard to performing required self-care actions when

1. Universal self-care is required under the usual conditions of the person's thermal environment?
2. Internal heat-regulating controls are disturbed?
3. External conditions affect body temperature?

rements for ources →

C. What other factors are present which would interfere with premotor, motor, or evaluative activities?

1. Emotional states
2. Pathologic conditions--physiologic or psychologic
3. Effects of drugs, activity limitations or other health-or disease-related measures

↓ Self-Care Action Abilities and Limitations ↓

↓

Nursing Requirements

self-care data – case material – reflects the belief of the Group about the type of research methodology that is most appropriate for empirical investigation in relation to self-care agency. It is also the belief of the Group that case study ma-

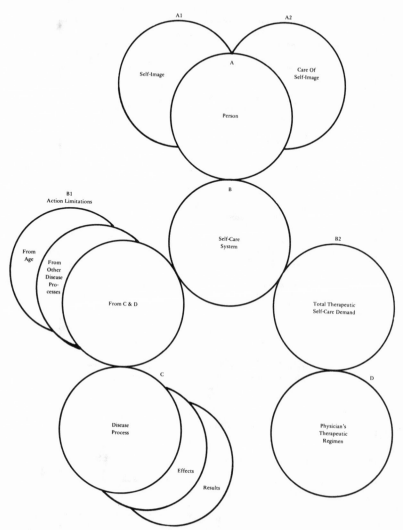

Figure 6-7 Framework to assess self-care agency in the presence of disease.

terial collected in the natural setting is crucial to the establishment of sound knowledge about self-care practices of persons or groups and is conditional for the valid use of experimental research.

A second outcome from the activities of the Group has been the *amplification of understanding of the underlying*

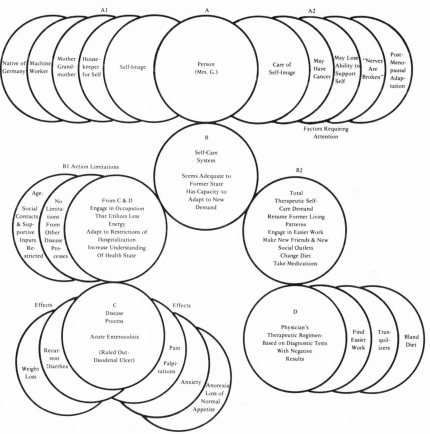

Figure 6-8   Example of assessment of self-care agency of a patient.

concepts that form the substantive structure of the concept of self-care agency. Complexities, such as the following, have been described:

1. Four types of self-care practices — universal self-care, universal self-care as modified by a health deviation, self-care resulting from a health deviation, and self-care resulting from therapy introduced to treat a health deviation
2. Social, cultural, and psychologic factors that influence self-care practices, including image of self as self-care practitioner, capacity to symbolize, linkage between systems of daily living and self-care systems, and cultural and scientific sources of health-related knowledge
3. Health state as a source of limitations of self-care agency

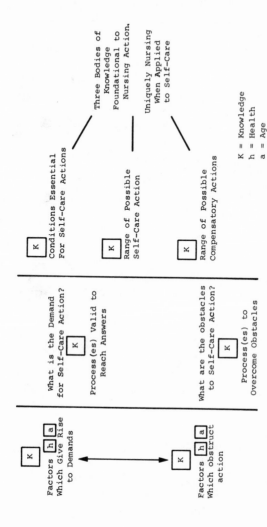

Figure 6-9 Areas of knowledge foundational to nursing action. Key: k = knowledge, h = health, a = age.

In addition, *distinctions* have been made between the terms *self-care deficit* and *self-care limitations,* which had been used interchangeably to describe self-care behaviors not adequate for required self-care. The distinction emerged during the meeting (August, 1970) in which models were drawn showing the concepts and relationship within the elements self-care agency, therapeutic self-care demand, and nursing agency. This work was a beginning formalization of the substantive structure of nursing. *Self-care limitation was accepted as one of the two elements in the substantive structure of self-care agency. Self-care deficit was accepted as expressive of the qualitative or quantitative inadequacy of self-care agency as related to therapeutic self-care demand.*

In the process of identification of the substantive structure underlying the concept of self-care agency, *several types of conceptual difficulties emerged in the Group,* all of which have implications for selection of the reality phenomena symbolized in the term. The *first conceptual problem* is the distinction of the system of self-care behaviors from the effects and cumulative results of utilizing that system. As defined in the previous chapter, self-care agency is the power of the person to engage in self-care behaviors; the product resulting from the use of those powers is the system of self-care behaviors. The self-care system produces results that can be described in relation to health state. The self-care behaviors (such as the behaviors involved in the selection, organization, preparation, and ingestion of nutritional elements) and the power to engage in these behaviors are the referents of the terms *self-care* and *self-care agency.* The effects on the health state of the individual (his nutritional status) are not in the substantive structure symbolized by the terms used in their most general sense.

The *second conceptual difficulty* is the establishment of a boundary between self-care and health-related self-care. Individuals engage in a system of daily living that relates to many components of human existence. The system of health-related self-care is a component of the system of daily living, but is not coexistensive with it. The NDCG has recognized

that the boundaries between the two concepts at present can
be drawn more easily and consistently in some areas of health-
related self-care than they can in others, for example, self-care
involving mental health. The mechanisms to deal with this
conceptual problem are limited by the instability of the related concept, mental health.

The *third conceptual problem* involves the mechanism for
integrating certain assumptions into the concept, self-care
agency. The assumptions are that self-care is deliberate or
voluntary behavior and that self-care may involve habit. Implicit in the concept is an acceptance of the following positions: Actions that are voluntary at some point in time may
become habitual; habitual actions may become the focus of
voluntary behavior; and individuals may not readily recall
the purpose or expected effects of actions that they perpetually
perform. This problem of symbolization has implications for
the specificity and consistency of the secondary elements
incorporated within the concept. It also has implications for
the selection of research methodologies that will accurately
locate the data necessary to investigate self-care behavior.

The *fourth conceptual problem* involves establishing boundaries to the concept along the dimension of the therapeutic
quality of the self-care behavior. The question involved here
is: Is behavior self-care even when it does not contribute in a
positive way to the health state? The concept of self-care
used by the Group does not include the assumption that the
self-care behavior contributes in reality in a positive way to
the health state. It does assume that at some point in time
the individual incorporated the action into his repertoire of
behaviors with the understanding that it was related to health
or well-being.

Although the establishment of boundaries of the concept
of self-care at times was and is a problem to individual members, it is important to recognize that there has been no
variation from the substance of the concept since the inception of the Group. Subsequent Group effort has refined
terminology and increased the members' depth of understanding of the substantive structure of this element of the con-

cept of nursing and of the concept of nursing system.

The effect of the activities engaged in by the Group over time is reflected in the model self-care agency (Fig. 6-10), which diagrams the network of elements and relationships that constitutes the substantive structure of self-care agency as perceived by the Group in 1970 [7].

Therapeutic Self-Care Demand

Therapeutic self-care demand has been *an integral theme* in the work of validating Orem's concept of nursing since the inception of the Group, but *its formalization as a concept took place during a period of three years.* The use of the term as a specific symbol for the theme emerged in the process of formalization. The activities of the Group in relation to this element of the concept of nursing again reflect the effort that is needed to isolate the substantive structure of a broad conceptual element of a general concept.

In the set of propositions about self-care presented at the initial meeting of the Nursing Model Committee, three general purposes for self-care are identified: continued existence; maintenance and promotion of health; and, in the event of disease, injury, or malfunctioning, the sustaining of life and the improvement of health. Another proposition explicitly states that "self-care which is directed to the maintenance and promotion of health requires a scientifically derived fund of knowledge about self-care goals and practices as well as related skills and habits."

The theme underlying this material points to *a source external to the individual from which requirements for self-care practices are derived.* At this point in Group thinking the description of therapeutic self-care was phrased *subjectively.* It was conceptualized as a quality of the abilities or capacities of the self-care agent. This orientation reflects the emphasis on self-care conduct that was dominant at the time.

The term *self-care demands* began to be used during the period (1966–1967) when the Group was analyzing patient data to validate the premises about self-care. The material at hand made it quite evident that the stimulus for self-care did

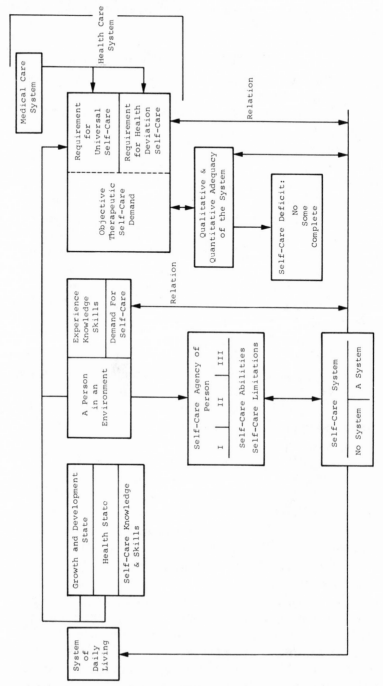

Figure 6-10 Self-care agency. Key: I = growth and developmental
state; II = integrated human functioning and purposive behaviors;
III = structure of person's self-care knowledge, developed self-care
skills.

not always arise within the patient, and in some of these instances the "demands," whether of internal or external origin,
did not seem to be necessarily therapeutic. The film reviewed
by the Group seems to have been a powerful demonstration
of this; the term *self-care demands* occurs more frequently
after the analysis of the film. Minutes began to make references
to "demands for therapeutic self-care."

The term *therapeutic self-care demand* as a *singular entity
reflecting a complement of requirements* represents *a refinement and abstraction in the level of thinking about self-care.*
Therapeutic self-care demand is grounded in the *objectively*
established need for engagement in self-care practices while
self-care agency is related to an existing behavioral repertoire.

This evolution has been accompanied by a corresponding
change in emphasis about the base for definition of the demand. Formerly, use of scientific knowledge as the base for
self-care was the primary criterion for application of the
label therapeutic. In this conceptualization, primary emphasis
is placed on interlinking of scientific knowledge with factors
inherent in the person and his environment (including those
that are culturally derived) to arrive at the combination that
can be judged as contributory to the promotion of health
and well-being.

Two activities the Group engaged in over time reflect the
position of the concept therapeutic self-care demand as an
element in the concept of nursing and indicate its relationship to the concept self-care agency. Through the Nursing
Model Committee *groups of nurses in specialty areas,* such
as medical-surgical nursing and psychiatric–mental health
nursing, *set forth statements identifying the proper object
and the subject matter content of their areas.* The statements
explicitly link the types of nursing to the therapeutic self-
care demands relevant to categories of patients. The statements are in the nature of generalizations about relationships
of categories of nurses and populations of patients grouped
by health deviation (except for the statement from public
health) and, where possible, by regularities or constancies

in known characteristics of self-care agency. The latter can be expressed as a generality only to the degree that characteristics of the population are known or that limitations are derivable from the known health state. The *relationship between nursing and the predictable therapeutic self-care demand* is represented in these statements.

The following are two examples of the statements submitted by groups of faculty:

Psychiatric Nursing — The object of psychiatric nursing is persons whose perceptions and behaviors may tend to be growth restrictive and divisive rather than growth promoting and unifying for self and others and consequently have demands for and limitations in therapeutic self-care. We feel that the type of assistance the nurse gives is in examining, evaluating, and modifying patterns of (a) experiencing inner and outer reality, and (b) relating to things, people, and events within a family group and as a member of the larger community.

DISTINCTIVE AREAS OF NURSING FUNCTION
1. The nurse works directly with the needs of the patient or in close relation to the total living situation.
2. The nurse provides for direct need-fulfillment: physiological, interpersonal, and sociocultural insofar as the patient is incapable of self-care.
3. The nurse functions on a basis of a holistic philosophy in assessing the areas of need and identifying and utilizing resources for need fulfillment.[2]

Public Health Nursing — The object of Public Health Nursing is the health of a neighborhood, a local, state, national, or international community, with focus on prevention of disease and disability, promotion and maintenance of health, and comprehensive care of the sick and disabled as this can be accomplished through assisting communities toward self-care, which contributes to the above.[3]

The *second activity* was the development by the NDCG of models to guide in the analysis of the effects and results of

---

[2] Presented to the Committee by C. Tuohey and M. A. Schroeder; developed by them in collaboration with Sr. Kathleen Black.

[3] Developed and presented to the Committee by Edna Solomon.

health states of individuals about whom case data had been collected. These models provide *a method of sorting out, in specific cases or in specific types of health conditions, what are the sources of the requirements for self-care and what is the nature of the total therapeutic self-care demand on a person arising from one's health condition.* These models indicate the distinction between self-care agency and therapeutic self-care demand. They also demonstrate that the latter serves to define the requisite state of the former at some point in time.[4]

This relationship between therapeutic self-care demand and self-care agency in the structure of the concept of nursing system provides a natural base for *a combination of research methodologies* for empirical exploration: *hypothetical-deductive method and case method.* The hypothetical-deductive method is applicable to exploration of some of the major influences determining therapeutic self-care demand in categories of patients. It is also of value in the initial determination of simulated effects of variations in self-care agency on meeting the demand.

The case method is especially useful in describing the summation of requirements of specific persons and self-care systems in relation to the therapeutic self-care demand. Case material and existing models are available to Group members for further development and for structuring knowledge about therapeutic self-care demand.

The *process of achieving conceptual consistency in the use of the term therapeutic self-care demand required more time than did the process related to self-care agency. One* of the major factors is that *the clustering of elements in the concept therapeutic self-care demand is an abstraction* that does not represent a specific, single, real-world event or a series of real-world events that concretely cluster together. *The individual who utilizes the term conceptually constructs the cluster.*

[4] Figures 6-7 and 6-8 are examples of these models.

The *problems* that appeared in the *members' utilization of the symbol* related to the identification of real-world phenomena that could accurately be admitted as relevant.

The *first problem* involved identification of the source from which the definition of the demand might flow. The word *therapeutic* carried the connotation that the demand is derived from medical science or results from a health deviation that exists in the individual. Thus interpreted, therapeutic self-care demand would be constituted from only a portion of the self-care requirements. The definition presented in this work indicates that the requirements derive from the objectively derived design of the purposive actions projected as instrumentally productive of positive health results for the individual. The conceptual problem relates to the ability to operate on the broadest interpretation of the term *therapeutic.*

The *second problem* involved the extent of the action component symbolized by the term. As defined here, the term is a symbol for a complex of requirements and the actions to be taken in meeting them, the totality being referred to as "the demand." In observation and analysis of case data, single actions or complexes of actions meeting a single need are readily discernible as being components of the therapeutic self-care demand. Communication shorthand often results in referring to these actions as the demand. Prolonged use of this pattern can lead to a change in the conceptual structure within individuals. The *conceptual problem involves retaining awareness of the totality of the framework even though the totality of real-world referents may not be accessible or evident.*

The *third problem* involved the accurate identification of data descriptive of the referents of the concept in the reality setting. Specifically, it related to *distinguishing the doing of the action from the demand.* The behaviors in the self-care system reflect the individual's perception of what the self-care demand is, but by themselves these behaviors are not accurate evidence of the therapeutic self-care demand. *The demand is in the nature of an information input to the individual; the self-care system is the action output that occurs in response.* Health sciences, as evident in medical science and in culture, are the sources in terms of which the therapeutic self-care demand can be defined.

The culmination of group thinking about the concept therapeutic self-care demand is included in Figure 6-10, Self-care agency, developed in 1970.

Nursing Agency

In the Group process up to 1970, which led to the development of the NDCG definition of nursing, *nursing agency as a term had not been introduced,* although the terms *nursing* and *nursing action* had been used continuously. The efforts of the Group to express their beliefs about nursing and to define the components of nursing action are a reflection of the difficulty that arises when individuals attempt to set forth the underpinnings of an integral component of their actions. In the Nursing Model Committee much of the focus of attention was on the elements, self-care agency and therapeutic self-care demand. On the whole there were *two trends of thinking about nursing* apparent in the Group during this period. First, *members tended to view situations and to speak as nurses.* The position they spoke from would more often be that of the *nurse conceptualizing the setting* than of the *conceptual theorist looking at nursing.* Second, *more emphasis was placed on the implications of self-care agency and therapeutic self-care demand for nursing than on the relationship of these elements within a concept of nursing.*

The *initial activity of the Group* in relation to what later became a concept of nursing agency involved a *critical examination of existing concepts of nursing.* The Group reviewed some premises about nursing that described the nature of nursing in relation to society and that had been developed by one of the members (Orem). Various conceptualizations of nursing, as presented in the literature by nursing theorists,[5] were discussed and the elements within them were compared. No formal decision was made by the Group about the accep-

[5] Faye Abdellah, Virginia Henderson, Dorothy Johnson, Bertrand Meyer, Loretta Heidgerken, Frances Reiter, Marguerite Kakosh, Ernestine Wiedenbach.

tance of any of these, but there was a subsequent move to explore the implications of the Orem premises about nursing.

SOME PREMISES ABOUT NURSING
1. Nursing is social action.
2. Nursing is a helping or assisting service.
3. Nursing is health service; its results are contributory to the continuation of rational life and to health maintenance and promotion.
4. Nurses accomplish life- and health-related results for persons by the application of scientifically derived knowledge and by the use of valid technologies to overcome self-care action deficits of persons which arise from situations of health in order to meet specific requirements for continuing or periodic self-care [8].

Of focal concern was the first premise, "nursing is social action," and *the point of inquiry* raised was *what was the nature of the unit act which occurred between nurse and patient and what conditions lead to variation in assignment of responsibility for its accomplishment.* The focus, thus, was interpersonal and not social in the fullest meaning of the term. Discussion topics which served as the modality for this inquiry were nursing the conscious and the unconscious patient, types of assisting actions in nursing, differences in the actions of nurse and patient when different types of patients are involved.

Although analytical exploration was more oriented to the identification of descriptions of the patient, some dimensions of nursing agency were established. Two categories of nurse behaviors, *observing and assisting,* were identified as essential in nursing a patient. Nursing action was viewed as the use of valid assisting technologies, selected for their appropriateness to a particular nursing situation. The range of forms of assisting actions in nursing was accepted as: doing for, teaching, guiding, supporting, and creating a developmental environment. The *range of forms of assisting actions was validated through use of patient data and the film review, previously described.*

The direction that Group effort took reflected the effects of a related activity undertaken simultaneously in the Group, *the exploration of action theory and its relevance for description of the nursing situation.* Figure 6-11 is a presentation of one of the models that emerged from the Nursing Model Committee in May, 1965.

At the conclusion of this phase of exploration (1967) not much movement had occurred in the formal expression of ideas about nursing agency. The statement of Premises about Nursing included in the 1967 Report of the Nursing Model Committee [9] contains relatively few changes in the statement set forth in 1965.

During the *second phase* of development (1968–1970),[6] *cognitive expression about nursing moved from the level of nursing related to a specific patient to the level of generalization about nursing.* The activity that seems to have been instrumental in this process was the previously described one in which specialty nursing groups defined the proper object and the subject matter of their areas. In this exercise, *nursing became the key element for cognitive organization and the outcome was a series of generalized statements about nursing in the specialty areas.* Movement into this phase began with the 1968 Report of the Nursing Model Committee, the terminal report of that Committee. In it can be found the first formal expression by the Group of the concept of nursing system. It reads:

A Nursing System is a complex action system formed by linking one or a combination of the ways of assisting to a patient self-care system or to some component part of the system. Nursing systems are designed to: (a) achieve patient health or health related goals through self-care which is therapeutic, (b) overcome self-care deficits, and (c) foster and preserve self-care abilities of the patient [10].

This statement identifies the link between valid ways of assisting (which is the nursing action) and the state of the patient self-care system.

In subsequent sessions, references to nursing action retain this context although the system terminology does not recur

[6]The terminal period of the Nursing Model Committee and the initial two years of the NDCG.

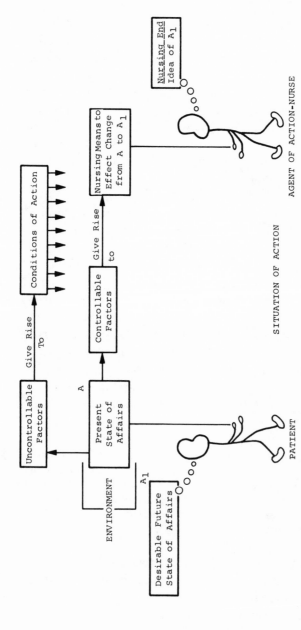

Figure 6-11 Parsons' elements of social action applied in a general way to nursing.

until later. The format for expression continued to be in the *form of tentative generalizations* (nursing will require . . .) *more often than conclusions about specific patients* even when patient situations were being discussed. The references also indicate that the actions performed by the nurse are selected from a range of actions of which the nurse is capable.

The developmental change most apparent during this period was in the *identification of the complexity of factors that affect the nursing situation and of which nurses must be aware.* Recognition was given to the fact that the link between nurse and patient arises between persons in a shared environment, each of whom exists in other environments. When the nursing process occurs, the nurse must take into account other environments in which the patient exists, for example, "the complexity of the nursing situation will vary according to the complexity of relevant communication networks" already existing between patient–physician–family [11].

Despite the fact that changes are apparent in the level of conceptualization about nursing actions, it should be noted that *only a small portion of the discussions during 1968 and 1969 focused directly on nursing actions.* None of the models during this period had nursing as their subject matter. The need to develop models indicating the nature of nursing agency was recognized under agenda items labelled "future work" but it was *not until 1970 that nursing actions and nursing systems became more central issues for Group discussion.*

An *essential question* implicit in the efforts to conceptualize nursing agency is the *relationship between a system and the boundaries.* The relationship can be viewed from two perspectives: (1) the effect of the environment on the nature of the system, or (2) the nature of the boundary distinguishing the system from its environment. In Group discussion attention tended to be centered on the environmental effects rather than on the boundaries. The fact that boundaries were being established to the concept of nursing system was not recognized and, consequently, the problem of the boundaries of the concept recurred later. The system-boundary problem, which recurred so frequently in Group discussion, is also reflective of the nature of the system under study. Buckley [12] has made the observation that the more open the system and the more highly flexible its structure, the more arbitrary are the distinctions between the boundaries and the environment. He comments that the source of the distinction is dependent in part on the purpose of the observer.

Engagement in the process of boundary establishment had an effect on the developing concept of nursing agency: The complexity of the action requirement on the nurse in *observation* increased and the *assisting* actions were tailored to more specific dimensions. In addition, another quality was identified as an essential within the range of nursing agency: the ability to *design* a system of nursing. This was seen as an intermediary between observing and assisting.

In the *third phase* in Group development (1970–1971) *nursing agency became the focus of effort. Nursing agency was located in a position within the concept of nursing system; nursing system assumed primacy as the organizing theme.* This phase began when the model of a nursing system (Fig. 6-12) was introduced as an abstraction from the discussion of the care of one patient [13]. The model makes explicit the nature of the linking system and also points to the determination of nursing action dependent on the values assigned to the patient self-care system and the therapeutic self-care demand.

The outcome of the effort expended during the previous years was expressed in a series of statements about nursing and the focus of nursing [14]. This work included a revision and elaboration of the premises accepted in 1965 (see p. 156). The first three premises were accepted as originally stated; the fourth premise was edited for clarification; a fifth, an additional premise, gave recognition to the fact that the recipient of nursing might be an individual, a small group (e.g., a family), or a large group (e.g., a community).

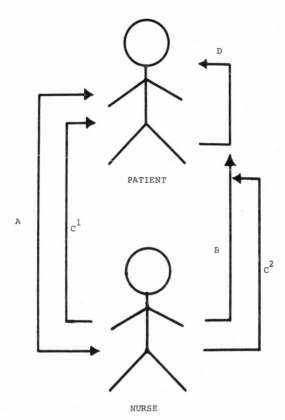

Figure 6-12   A partly compensatory system of nursing. Key: A = the interpersonal situation, interactions, and techniques to initiate, maintain, and sever interpersonal relationships. B = set of technologies for assisting the patient to overcome self-care limitations. C^1 = health-care techniques directed toward the patient or the environment. The nurse is in the role of agent. C^2 = techniques to assist the patient in the role of agent. D = patient as a self-care agent.

The other materials that were produced viewed nursing from a variety of perspectives reflecting the depth that had developed in Group thinking about nursing. Materials included statements about the proper object of nursing, the focus of the process of nursing, and new premises about nursing. These are presented with minor revisions.

I. Proper Object of Nursing: The object of nursing is a person or a group of persons with inabilities to provide or manage self-care of a therapeutic quality.

II. Focus of the Process of Nursing: The process of nursing has a dual focus on the *person as agent* and on *categories of techniques* related to or derived from: the specific focus(es) of health care for the person; universal self-care to maintain life and health; and the person living with a health problem(s) and its effects and with therapy and its effects.

III. Premises about Nursing as a Discipline
   A. Nursing is a practice discipline.
   B. Nursing as a body of knowledge incorporates scientific findings about deliberate actions and health as well as the technologies related to health care, self-care, and ways of assisting.
   C. Nursing in its practical aspect includes process and art.
   D. The nursing process includes
      1. The identification of (a) the demands for self-care action, (b) the obstacles to a patient's performance of the required self-care actions, (c) the self-care deficit
      2. The design and control of a system of nursing assistance in light of 1a, b, and c
      3. Planning for the delivery of nursing and providing nursing according to the design of the system and in the light of changing conditions in the patient or the environment of the patient
   E. The art of nursing is a quality resulting from a blend of the nurse's talents, personality, and knowledge, which enable the nurse to create the design of a nursing system or some component of a nursing system for a particular patient and to translate the design into nursing action.

These 1970 statements reflect the thinking of the Group in relation to the nature of nursing in society, the factors affecting nursing, and techniques involved in the nursing process. They set forth most explicitly the relationship of the art and the process of nursing.

Three terms were in common usage up to this point: *nursing, nursing process,* and *nursing system.* It was characteristic of Group discussions to use these inconsistently. At times they were used interchangeably and at times distinctly. Concurrently, it was an accepted belief that not all the potential action capacities of a nurse were brought into play in a specific nursing situation. *Nursing agency as a term* was introduced into the spectrum during the 1970 period of Group activity. It was accepted as the power of the nurse to engage in nursing actions (observation, design, and assistance). The *relationship* of the *four terms to each other came into conscious perspective only after the development of the concept of nursing systems with its elements.*

Only a few Group exercises have focused on examination of nursing agency. However, individually, *members have engaged in a variety of studies* that have contributed to thought on this point. These studies have, for the most part, been exploratory and descriptive in nature. All have as their *focus* the *translation of nursing agency into specific nursing actions.* Two different organizing themes are apparent in the studies. One builds initially on generalizations about the nature of the therapeutic self-care demand and secondarily on the nature of the self-care system, especially on predictable changes in the nature of the self-care system resulting from the medical therapy. The second builds primarily on self-care capacities and limitations and secondarily on the nature of the therapeutic self-care demand in various situations.

In the *first type,* there are *two modes* for organization of the problem in relation to nursing agency. *One approach* has focused on the *identification of the range of nursing actions for case loads of patients:* the ambulatory diabetic, the ambulatory cardiac patient taking sodium warfarin, the patient having gynecologic surgery, the obstetric patient. In these studies the nature of the health state, the process for delivery of health care, and the predictable concerns of patients with that health condition are established as the dimensions influencing the requirements for nursing agency at various points in time.

The *second approach* has focused on the *identification of the range of nursing actions related to specific components of medical therapy,* such as administration of medications or performance of procedures. In this approach, the conditions essential to the process and the steps of the process form the dimensions determining nursing agency.

In both approaches it is possible to determine the nature of nursing agency that must be present in the nurses who enter the situation. It is also possible to set some determinations on the components of nursing agency that will be activated under various conditions, although it is implicit that the final determination occurs when the dimensions and results of the existing self-care system of a patient can be described.

The *second type of study* focuses on *identification of categories of factors affecting self-care capacities of patients*. In this type of study, the range of nursing actions is considered in relation to the range of existing capacities in patients (communication, cognitive operations, ability to function in complex settings), which in turn must be seen in relation to the therapeutic self-care demand on the patient.

In this type of study, it is possible to determine the nature of nursing agency that must be present in the nurses and to define some of the specific factors involved in assessment of the self-care system.

Both types of studies reflect the belief of the Group about the nature of empirical work necessary for the establishment of a well-grounded nursing science. Research endeavors need to be directed toward the identification of the factors that help define the interaction link that constitutes the nursing system in a specific situation; more detailed exploratory and hypothetical deductive effort must precede experimental study. Research involving the creation of an end product, in this case an effective nursing system, is a vital component in this development.

When nurses engage in discussions about nursing or patients, a common phrase is, "It is hard to generalize because every patient is so individual." In the operational situation, generalizations must be incorporated into a system of delivery of nursing care that takes into account many specific factors about the patient and the environment. *Nurses have more awareness of the need to adapt to specificity than they do of the extent of the generalities they utilize in practice situations.*

The process, which the NDCG members have engaged in since the inception of the Group in 1965, is one of abstracting and labeling the underpinnings of nursing operations.

Several different types of problems have been apparent as members moved toward making explicit, or developing, their conceptual structure of nursing and nursing agency. One related to *the tendency to organize descriptions around patients as individuals* rather than on *the actions each patient and nurse performed in health care.* The emphasis on individuals focused thinking at the specific level. The focus that developed in the Group was on the action component of behavior. This variation, if followed through to its consequences, brings forth a different ordering of data and a different clustering of categories from that derived when the "patient as individual" is the organizing component.

The *second distinction* that the present definition of nursing system calls for *is one that must be made between the assisting action and the interpersonal relationship.* When nursing is viewed primarily as an interpersonal relationship, it is difficult to retain awareness of the purpose of the relationship. The definition of nursing system places emphasis on nursing as assistance with the recognition that accomplishment requires that an effective interpersonal relationship be maintained. Related to this distinction is the requirement for conceptualization of the accomplishment of assisting actions through the coordination of specific actions of more than one person.

A *third conceptual problem* that was evident again focused on the *establishment of some system for evaluating the reality behaviors of the nurse.* Observations of the behavior of nurses in practice situations often produce evidence that more time is spent in coordination of activities in a health-care setting than in care of patients. *Analysis of reality situations can proceed from the perspective of the proper object of each discipline or from the perspective of the reality behaviors of persons occupying various positions.* In the activities of the NDCG greater emphasis was placed on the former mode of operation and on the structuring of reality situations in light of the outcome.

The *fourth conceptual problem* that was closely linked to

the problem of defining system boundaries *involved the emphasis placed on autonomy of nursing actions and coordination of nursing actions with those of others.* The problem involves the abstraction of a framework to establish the relationship between these actions and thereby to derive the organization of services. The points of difference return to the question of whether the proper object or the number of reality demands is the source of the definition.

This 1971 synthesis of the concept of nursing agency drew the concept into a perspective in relation to self-care agency and therapeutic self-care demand and it established a framework for use of the terms *nursing, nursing agency, nursing process,* and *nursing system.* The summary of this work is presented in Figure 6-13.

Summary, 1965–1971

This summary of Group process over time indicates the efforts made to establish a conceptual structure that has some degree of validity and reliability. The development of dominant themes is a process of successive abstraction and generalization that has been dynamic and has established certain boundaries within the reality situation.

As a dynamic process, the exploration of the elements in the concept has led to more specific descriptions and more accurate conceptualizations. The initial focus of the Group was on a patient, a nurse, and their relationship to each other. The product at this point represents an abstraction that symbolizes the action linkages leading to action output rather than the persons involved. The characteristics of the person who participates in the action are seen as attributes affecting the quality and quantity of that component of the action system. The system itself is the combination of self-care action and assisting action. The work of development of the substantive structure of the elements has resulted in a more accurate conceptualization of factors that affect legitimate occupancy of statuses of nurse and patient in a nursing system.

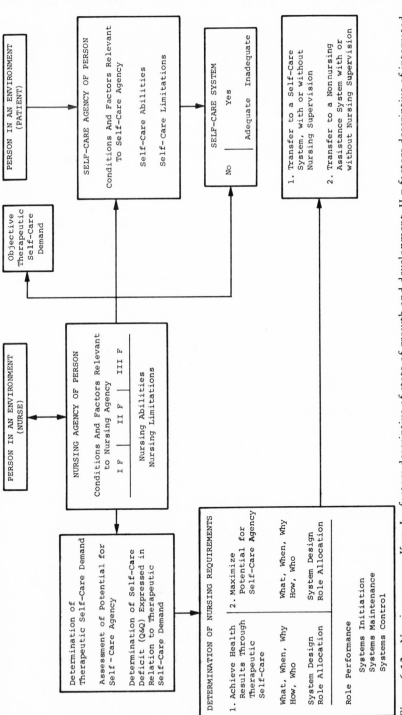

Figure 6-13 Nursing agency. Key: I = factors descriptive of state of growth and development. II = factors descriptive of integrated human functioning as it relates to purposive behavior. III = structured nursing knowledge and nursing performance abilities.

A *nurse's legitimate patient* is one of whom it can be said:

1. This individual, with subsets of self-care agency and therapeutic self-care demand, requires nursing because of some health-related self-care deficits.
2. The areas in which this individual validly requires assistance are in specific a, b, c aspects of therapeutic self-care demand because his self-care agency in these aspects of care is limited in definite x, y, z ways.

The *legitimate occupant of the status, nurse,* is one of whom it can be said: The nurse, with the subset of nursing agency, has knowledge of, and ability to use, ways of identifying patient health-derived or health-related self-care deficits, ways of assisting the patient to overcome self-care deficits, and ways of designing, initiating, maintaining, and regulating nursing systems.

As a boundary process, the development of the elements in the general concept has established a limit between the nursing system and its environment. The Group has given recognition to the fact that the nursing system and the persons in it are located in an environment that influences both the system and its occupants. Formalization of the concept made it possible to establish priorities and contingencies in the discussion of generalizations and of real-world phenomena. Although the concept affords this possibility, the maintenance of consistent boundaries is in part the responsibility of the individual's own thought processes.

During the exploration of the elements and relationship between them, the nursing system itself was accepted as the independent unit for analysis. The maintenance of the nursing system in this priority position was difficult and was the source of repeated discussions and disagreements among members. As stated and described here, it is not readily apparent that the concept includes recognized linkages to other health disciplines, especially not beyond the physician.

Although the questions of formalization of ideas and of boundaries are closely linked to each other, the Group was not able to deal with both simultaneously. Emphasis was placed on the formalization of the general concept. Only when this was accomplished were members of the Group in a position to explore consistently the location of other linkages, such as those to other health-care personnel, within the relationship structure specified by the concept.

Utilization of the concept, in discussion or in observation of real-world phenomena, requires that the user maintain a mental framework sufficiently abstract to account for the variations of real-world phenomena that might exist, but yet sufficiently specific to allow discrimination of relevant items of data. Concept utilization in areas such as nursing requires ability to engage in transpositions of thought processes. The stimulus for calling the concept into operation may be a specific event in the concrete order. The ultimate product may appear as an event in the concrete order. The quantity and quality of the actions of the nurse in the linking process are reflective of the knowledge base upon which the nurse draws and of the intellectual operations the nurse must engage in to produce effective nursing systems.

BASIC CONDITIONING FACTORS

The further development of the patient variables expressed in the 1970 general concept of nursing system was continued during the period 1972 to 1974 and thereafter. One development was the identification and analysis of factors that were judged to have an active influence at points in time on the concrete values of the *therapeutic self-care demand* or the *self-care agency* of individuals. From a *nursing systems* perspective these factors could be considered as the *parameters* of the *patient variables.*[7]

Eight Factors

During the period 1972 to 1974 the NDCG members through their work in nursing practice situations or in the analysis of case material accepted eight factors that affected the values of the patient variables at points in time. The term used by

[7] It was recognized that the parameters of the patient variables also functioned as parameters of the nurse variable, nursing agency. However, at this time the focus of attention and inquiry was the patient variables.

Group members to refer to these factors is *basic conditioning factors.* The eight factors, some of which are intrinsic to individuals, are listed.

1. Age
2. Sex
3. Developmental state
4. Health state
5. Sociocultural orientation
6. Health care system elements (e.g., medical diagnostic and treatment modalities)
7. Family system elements
8. Patterns of living

All of the basic conditioning factors had been identified by and worked with during the period 1958 to 1971 by Orem in relation to the *self-care requirements* of patients and their *abilities* and *limitations* for engagement in self-care [15]. The NDCG's attention to these factors grew out of the need of Group members in practice situations to determine the values of the two patient variables at points in time. This required the determination of conditioning effects of age, sex, developmental state, and other factors on the patient's therapeutic self-care demand and self-care agency. Attention to the factors also resulted from the awareness on the part of Group members in nursing education of the need for (1) organizing knowledge about the conditioning effects of the eight factors on the universal self-care requirements, and (2) the articulating of nursing with the sciences of man and the medical sciences.

The beginning and growing conceptualizations of Group members about the nature and functions of *basic conditioning factors* with respect to the *therapeutic self-care demand* and *self-care agency* increased the ability of members to deal with the complexity of concrete complementary elements in concrete situations of practice in their design and production of nursing systems. As insights about the functions of basic conditioning factors increased, so did the Group members' understanding of how to sort out and relate patient data in nursing practice situations as well as their understanding of points of articulation of the subject matter of nursing with subject matter descriptive and explanatory of the eight factors. It should be understood that the attention of the NDCG from the point of view of inquiry was focused on the technological component of nursing systems as described in Chapter 5. Members understood that all or some of the eight factors would affect both the interpersonal and social components of nursing systems also identified in Chapter 5.

The work of individual NDCG members and Group deliberations resulted in the formulation and expression of a definition of a basic conditioning factor at the October 5, 1974, meeting of the NDCG [16]. *Basic conditioning factor* was defined as follows:

something which precipitates a chain of intrahuman events which may [change existent requirements] or bring about added requirements for deliberate regulatory inputs to the person or [the person's] environment or affect the value of self-care agency.

Conditioning Factors and Patient Variables

The basic conditioning factors are viewed not as explanatory of the structure of the patient variables but as conditioning their values at instants in time. For example, a given magnitude of age and developmental state does not explain self-care agency but it is a determinant of its stage of development and therefore of its value at points in time.

The basic conditioning factors have as their referents existent human conditions or ongoing series of events that exercise an active influence on identifiable human abilities (self-care agency), and human requirements (self-care requirements) within a time frame or affect the means that can be used to meet requirements. The number of basic conditioning factors, the magnitudes of which are changing rapidly, will increase the complexity of nursing practice situations [15, p. 53].

Known relationships between a conditioning factor and these human operations and requirements can be expressed as a conditional proposition.

Such conditional propositions are *laws* that express the interdependence between variable magnitudes of a basic conditioning factor and some values within the possible range of values of self-care agency or therapeutic self-care demand. Such laws when formulated would assert relations of "functional dependence" (function being used in the mathematical sense) between the conditioning factors and the patient variables [17].

The bases for many conditional propositions or laws expressing relations between the eight identified basic conditioning factors and the therapeutic self-care demand and the self-care agency of persons who can benefit from nursing are understood by experienced nurses. The formulation of laws expressing such relations would contribute substantially to the structuring of nursing knowledge and the advance of nursing science.

Basic System .

Early in the period when *basic conditioning factors* were the focus of attention of the NDCG members, the term *basic system* was introduced. The term emerged during a presentation to the Group of the results of a project conducted by five Group members to model the concrete dimensions of systems of nursing for a population of women with myomata uteri who were treated medically by surgical removal of the uterus. The term was used initially to express the reason for an individual or a population moving into an active patient status within a health-care system. The referent of *basic system* could be, for example, *a specific disease process, a specific mode of medical diagnosis or treatment,* or *a specific life cycle situation.*

The initial meaning attached to the term *basic system* by Group members reflected the Group's earlier development and use of what was referred to as the *basic approach model* for use in nursing practice situations. The model suggested that in initial contacts with patients nurses attend to the following:

1. The reason(s) for the person being under or seeking health care with attention to the relation of this to
   a. the patient's prior system of self-care
   b. the patient's value system
2. The interests and concerns of the patient
3. The patient's self-image
4. The effects and results of the events that caused the person to seek and be under health care. The nature of these effects and results could require that the nurse while working with the patient as *person* at the same time be able to think within a frame of reference of the patient as *agent* or *symbolizer* or *organism* or *object*.

The model was not a substitute for definitive nursing diagnostic endeavors but a means to help nurses orient themselves to patients coming under nursing care.

The use of the term *basic system* was later extended to refer to any one of the basic conditioning factors that was actively influencing the values of self-care agency or therapeutic self-care demand. The conclusion was that the factor that was operational in bringing an individual or a population to active patient status in a health care system should be investigated and understood in its relations to other basic systems that are actively influencing the values of self-care agency and therapeutic self-care demand.

The extension of the meaning of the term *basic system* brought into focus the need in nursing practice situations to identify the basic conditioning factors that in one or more of their concrete modalities were generating conditions or events within patients or their environments that were conditioning or could condition the values of patients' self-care agency or therapeutic self-care demand. For example, in the project on standard-setting for nursing systems for women with myomata uteri a number of basic systems were identified. These included the ones indicated below in relation to three basic conditioning factors.

BASIC CONDITIONING FACTORS

1. Sex

   Fact — Patients are women

BASIC SYSTEMS

1a. Life-giving, life-bearing, and mothering processes

1b. Sexual identity processes

2. Health State
   Fact — Health state is characterized by events associated with myomata uteri

   2a. Pathologic processes associated with the formation of myomata uteri
   2b. Associated pathologic events in structures adjacent to the uterus including the excretory organs

3. Health Care System Elements
   Medical treatment modalities
   Fact — Patients and their physicians have entered into an agreement for surgical removal of the uterus

   3a. Structural changes associated with the surgical removal of the uterus
   3b. Physiologic events associated with the surgical removal of the uterus
   3c. Psychologic and psychosocial events associated with
       (1) making the decision for surgical removal of the uterus
       (2) the surgical removal of the uterus
       (3) the effects and results of the removal of the uterus

The foregoing is offered as an example, not as an exhaustive laying out of the *basic systems* identified in the project from which the example is taken.

In group discussion, the value of using the term *basic system* was questioned. "Basic condition" and "basic factor" were suggested as substitutes. However, the use of the term continued. Group members who were in the process of moving a static concept of *basic conditioning factor* to a dynamic state perceived that the idea of *basic system* facilitated this process. As insights of the Group members about the basic conditioning factors increased, basic systems were thought of as specific modalities of the conditioning factors that were actively affecting the values of the patient elements of nursing systems.

The idea of *basic system* grew out of nursing practice situations. Thinking *basic system(s)* within nursing practice situations can be viewed as a cognitive component of *nursing agency* that serves the nurse in the sorting out of patient data and in moving data about specific basic conditioning factors into a nursing frame of reference. Understanding on the part of nurses of the specific modalities of the parameters of the nursing system variables and ability to make judgments about the degree to which one or a combination of them are affecting the values of self-care agency and therapeutic self-care demand are considered as essential for effective nursing practice.

Views of Man

During the period 1972 to 1974 and thereafter, the views of man that the NDCG members perceived as specific to nursing became a focus of Group discussion. These views are man as *person, agent, symbolizer, organism* and *object* subject to gravitational forces. Of particular interest to Group members was the relationship of the views of man to the patient variables of nursing systems and to the factors that condition their value.

Group deliberations took the form of discussions about these relationships and the development of models to show relationships (1) among the different views of man and (2) between the views of man and the patient variables of nursing systems on the one hand and their parameters on the other. In Group deliberations the relationships of views of man to specific disciplines of knowledge were recognized.

In the February 16, 1973 meeting members formalized and expressed the following tentative agreements.

1. Individuals in the health-care disciplines are interested in man as a unitary being but each discipline has its own special focus or focuses.
2. In nursing situations and depending on the reason why a *person* is under health care, the four special focuses may have a particular order (e.g. *agent, symbolizer, organism, object,* or *agent, object*).
3. In nursing situations priorities can be set in relation to the way the views of man are ordered (e.g., with an adult, ambulatory population the views of man that have priority for the nurse are *agent* and *symbolizer*).
4. The four special views of man named in item 2 have a place and time orientation and are conceptually related not only to thera-

peutic self-care demand and self-care agency but also to the basic conditioning factors operational in nursing systems.

5. Knowledge about the views of man specific to nursing would be drawn from (a) the sciences of man (e.g., human psychology, human anatomy and physiology), and (b) selected applied sciences (e.g., developmental psychology).

6. Three of the special views of man, namely, *agent, symbolizer,* and *organism* are related as a construct with the following form:

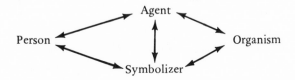

7. More specific views of man fit within the frame of reference provided by one or more of the four special views of man; for example, man as an "energy converter."

8. Particular basic conditioning factors that are actively affecting the values of self-care agency or therapeutic self-care demand would bring into operation in the nurse knowledge organized from the perspective of one or more of the special views of man. For example, when the health states of individuals are characterized by events associated with central nervous system disorders the views of man as *organism, agent,* and *symbolizer* sequentially came into operation within the thought processes of the nurse. This leads the nurse to the significant question: How will the patient as person be affected?

9. The views of man that are the special views of the discipline, nursing, are significant views for persons under nursing care as well as for nurses. These views come into operation within the thought processes of persons under nursing care when they begin to conceptualize *self* in a way that is meaningful for purposes of self-care including the development or management of their self-care agency.

10. Nurses' awareness of patients' abilities to *symbolize* self not only as *person* but also as *agent,* as *organism,* and as *object* is an important dimension of nursing practice.

Discussions focused on nursing's special *views of man* continued during Group meetings in 1973 and 1974. Questions with a focus on practice organized discussions; for example, when age is known to be functional as a parameter of the patient variables in a nursing system what view(s) of man does the nurse take? Other discussions were centered on the need for deliberate articulation of the medical and behavioral sciences with nursing.

The view of man as *organism* was the center of discussion in the February 16, 1974, meeting of five NDCG members. Consideration of the articulations of the subject matter of nursing with the biologic sciences with their focus on man as *organism* brought into consideration the role of knowledge of the biologic sciences in (1) the development or rehabilitation of the body image on the part of persons under health care, and (2) understanding on the part of individuals of the biologically oriented universal self-care requirements (e.g., maintaining an adequate intake of water).

During the February 16, 1974, meeting another focus of discussion was the biologic consideration of levels of organization including relationships of conceptualized parts to whole and whole to parts with a focus on both structural and functional dimensions. It was agreed that nurses should be able to differentiate between a general *organism* focus (a broad biologic functional focus — e.g., oxygenation of tissues) and an organ or a part approach. Either of these two focuses was considered as appropriate in nursing when nurses are attending to the biologic events characterizing an individual's health or developmental state.

During these deliberations a conceptual flow model was developed to indicate that when the nurse's thoughts are focused on a conceptualized part biologically described such as an organ or tissue or a cellular element, thinking should then move to a higher level of biologic organization and finally to the level of the organism considered as a structural and functional unity. It would be at this level that individuals considered as persons who are agents and symbolizers would be affected. It would also be at this level that individuals can be viewed as able or unable to control their position and movement in space and when *unable* the view of *man as object* would become operational in nurse or patient.

The biologic approach to *man as organism* was viewed as being in contrast to the *man as person in an environment* approach. It was agreed that nurses need to be able to use a combination of both approaches in nursing situations.

SUMMARY

The work of development of a conceptual structure for nursing that has some degree of validity and reliability encompassed the following as a first phase of development.

1. The development of the dominant themes (the broad conceptual structure) of the concept of nursing system expressed in the definition of nursing system (see Chap. 5). The focus here was on the technologic nursing system (see Fig. 5-1).
2. The formulation and expression of definitions of legitimate patient and legitimate nurse. The focus here was on the *social* components of the nursing system (see Fig. 5-1) defined in terms of the technologic components.
3. Through the foregoing and from a systems perspective establishing the limits between a nursing system and its environment.

In a second phase of development the broad conceptual elements within the expressed concept of nursing system were examined in relation to human and environmental factors that conditioned the values of these conceptual elements. Within a system frame of reference the patient variables (therapeutic self-care demand and self-care agency) were examined in relation to eight factors (parameters of the variables) that could condition the values of the variables at points in time. A specific parameter was referred to as a *basic conditioning factor* and, when concretely operational in one or more of its modalities, as a *basic system*.

The positing of a conditioning relation between the *eight factors* — age, sex, and so on — and *therapeutic self-care demand* and *self-care agency* contributed to the members' understanding of the conceptualized elements of nursing systems and their concrete referents.

The views of man accepted by the Group as special to nursing were examined in relation to both patient variables of nursing systems and the parameters of the variables. It was agreed that the views are related to both therapeutic self-care demand and self-care agency and to the eight basic conditioning factors. The views of man provide nurses with frames of reference to guide in using knowledge from a range of disciplines.

Results of continued work of the NDCG members that focused on the patient and nurse variables of nursing systems are presented in subsequent chapters.

REFERENCES

1. Nursing Model Committee.   Report to the Graduate Curriculum Committee of the School of Nursing (typewritten), The Catholic University of America, Washington, D.C., Apr. 20, 1967. P. 3.
2. Nursing Development Conference Group.   Minutes of the Nov. 1, 1969 Meeting (typewritten). P. 3.
3. Ashby, W. R.   The effect of experience on a determinate dynamic system. *Behav. Sci.* 1:35–42, 1956.
4. Hartnett, L. M.   Development of a theoretical model for the identification of nursing requirements in a selected aspect of self-care. The Catholic University of America, unpublished master's dissertation, 1968.
5. Nursing Development Conference Group.   Minutes of the Meeting of Oct. 4, 1968 (typewritten). Revised Nov. 16, 1968, July, 1971.
6. Nursing Development Conference Group.   Minutes of the Meeting of Mar. 21, 1970 (typewritten). Revised July, 1971.
7. Nursing Development Conference Group.   Minutes of the Meeting of Aug. 26–28, 1970 (typewritten).
8. Nursing Model Committee.   Minutes of the Meeting of Apr. 20, 1967 (typewritten). Also appears in the same form in the minutes of Apr. 26, 1965. P. 3.
9. Nursing Model Committee.   Minutes of the Meeting of May 20, 1967 (typewritten).
10. Nursing Model Committee.   Report to the Graduate Curriculum Committee, May 24, 1968 (typewritten). P. 3. Developed by Dorothea E. Orem Nov. 16, 1967, and revised by Committee members on May 10, 1968.
11. Nursing Development Conference Group.   Minutes of the Meeting of Aug. 1, 1969 (typewritten). P. 2.
12. Buckley, W.   *Sociology and Modern Systems Theory.* Englewood Cliffs, N.J.: Prentice-Hall, 1967. P. 3.
13. Nursing Development Conference Group.   Minutes of the Meeting of Feb. 21, 1970 (typewritten).

14. Nursing Development Conference Group. Minutes of the Meeting of Mar. 21, 1970 (typewritten). Pp. 2—3.
15. Orem, D. E. *Nursing: Concepts of Practice.* New York: McGraw-Hill, 1971. Pp. 51, 83.
16. Nursing Development Conference Group. Minutes of the Meeting of Oct. 5, 1974 (typewritten).
17. Nagel, E. *The Structure of Science.* New York: Harcourt, Brace & World, 1961. Pp. 56—57, 77—78.

7

Self-Care Agency: A Conceptual Analysis

THE CONCEPT

Self-care agency is the term that NDCG members use to refer to the *power* of individuals to engage in self-care. The term is a symbol for a human characteristic, a capability for a particular form of action (self-care). The capability begins to develop in childhood, attains a degree of perfection in adulthood, and declines with advancing age. *Agency* is used in the sense of "a means for exerting power," an "ability." The person who exercises this power can be referred to as the self-care agent or actor. The terms *agent* and *actor* are used within the frame of reference of action theory [1–5].

The conceptual construct *self-care agency* is utilized by NDCG members in two frames of reference. One frame of reference is that of *individual human beings* who are born into and grow, develop, and function within social groups and under a range of physical, biologic, and social environmental conditions. In this frame of reference self-care agency is thought of as a human characteristic. The second frame of reference is that of *nursing system* in which two patient variables, *self-care agency* and *therapeutic self-care demand,* are conceptualized as interactive with one nurse variable, *nursing agency* (Chap. 5, p. 107).

From a nursing perspective and a systems frame of reference, the two patient variables and the relationship between them set the specifications for nursing agency. From a self-care perspective, therapeutic self-care demand sets the specifications for self-care agency as well as for self-care (Chap. 5, p. 115). Within the frame of reference of *nursing system,* the cognitive operations of the nurse proceed according to the hypothetico-deductive mode. If an individual's *therapeutic self-care demand* has the value A and the person's *self-care agency* has the value B, and if B is not equal to A, then *nurs-*

181

ing agency should be operational according to specifications set by the values A and B including the relationship between them.

Self-care agency as a conceptual construct has been useful to NDCG members in nursing practice, in the exploratory stages of research, and in the structuring of nursing knowledge. To further the utility of the concept, NDCG members agree to the necessity of (1) the exposition of the domain and boundaries of a body of knowledge that would be descriptive and explanatory of self-care agency, and (2) an analysis of the structure of the concept self-care agency. These expositions are presented in two sections. The reality foundations for self-care agency expressed or implied in the premises and propositions about self-care (pp. 132–134), Hartnett's models of action (Figs. 6-1 through 6-5), and the NDCG members' understandings about deliberate action provided a general base for the work reported.

The presentations are made within a structured knowledge frame of reference with some identification of implications for nursing practice. The intent is to describe that which is or should be the object of nurses' attention in nursing practice. The significance of the concepts and ideas presented for nursing practice as well as for nursing research is evident. It is the formalization of the concepts and their organization into logical structures that is viewed by NDCG members as innovative and important for nursing. Mastery of even this nucleus of knowledge about self-care agency is viewed as essential for nurses' development and exercise of important perceptual and reasoning skills in nursing practice.

SELF-CARE AGENCY: AN AREA OF KNOWLEDGE
Scholars and theorists who engage in the endeavor of structuring knowledge around a specific concept such as self-care agency move from already developed insights about the entity to which inquiry is directed [6]. The 1973 NDCG model of self-care agency (Fig. 6-10) and the definition of self-care agency (see Chap. 5, p. 118) express some early in-

sights of members about self-care agency. Some of these insights considered for knowledge-building purposes are formulated and expressed as a set of propositions.

Eight Propositions About Self-Care Agency

1. Self-care agency is a complex, acquired human characteristic or quality.
2. Self-care agency is the power of an individual to engage in the operations essential for self-care.
3. The exercise by an individual of the power that is named self-care agency results in a system of actions directed to reality conditions in self or environment in order to regulate them; or its exercise results in a design and plan for such a system of action.
4. Self-care agency can be conceptualized as an action repertoire of an individual.
5. Self-care agency can be characterized in terms of abilities and limitations of an individual for engagement in self-care.
6. Conditions and factors in the environment of an individual affect the development of and the exercise of self-care agency.
7. Persons are subject to time sequential needs for the exercise of self-care agency.
   a. Knowledge about and awareness of internal conditions and external environmental conditions, the regulation of which requires self-care, constitute a need.
   b. Knowledge and awareness of a need to determine what internal and external conditions set up requirements for self-care constitute a need.
   c. Knowledge of what is in need of regulation at a given time combined with knowledge of effective regulatory measures constitutes a need.
   d. Judgments and decisions that specific regulatory measures should or will be used in the provision of self-care constitute a need.
   e. Initiation or continuation of self-care to achieve goals formulated in terms of regulation of known internal and external conditions constitutes a demand for continued exercise of self-care agency.
   f. Knowledge of the requisite to determine the effects and results of self-care constitutes a need.
8. Self-care agency is an estimative capability and a productive capability for self-care.

The foregoing propositions summarize some early positions taken by the NDCG members about *self-care agency* that gave direction to further inquiry.

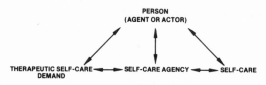

Figure 7-1   Boundary elements for a body of knowledge of self-care agency.

The subpropositions under the seventh proposition indicate that the *relationship* between the patient variable therapeutic self-care demand and the patient variable self-care agency can be expressed as a *need for exercise of.* However, the eighth proposition has implicit in it the idea that it is through the exercise of self-care agency that the therapeutic self-care demand is (1) determined (estimated) and known, and (2) met. Both propositions are based on the idea that the therapeutic self-care demand is a program of action.

One consideration of significance in knowledge building was the work of differentiation of the concept self-care from the concept self-care agency and the identification of the relationship between the two concepts. The NDCG members recognized early that working with these two concepts required thinking within a *person frame of reference* and not in an *organism frame of reference* [7]. They also recognized that thinking *self-care agency* required a mode of thought and a conceptual structure different from that required in thinking *self-care.* Four expressed concepts, *person, self-care agency, therapeutic self-care demand,* and *self-care,* and the relationships among them were recognized as setting limits for a body of knowledge about self-care agency (Fig. 7-1). The concepts named in the figure and the relationships among them are considered as a first delimitation of the domain of a body of knowledge about self-care agency.

A Hierarchy of Concepts
It is helpful in structuring knowledge around a concept to understand its relationships to more general and less general concepts (i.e., to locate a concept within a hierarchy of concepts) [8]. Figure 7-2 shows a schema for locating three of

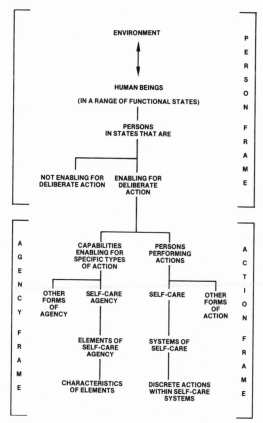

Figure 7-2   Three frames of reference, a hierarchical structuring of concepts.

the named concepts of Figure 7-1 within hierarchies. The named concepts so located constitute three frames of reference, namely, a person, an agency, and an action frame.

The most general and inclusive concept named in Figure 7-2 is "Human Beings" characterized *in a range of functional states;* individual human beings characterized as "persons" are *divided* into the logical categories of persons in states that *are enabling for* and *not enabling for* engagement in deliberate action. Persons in the former category are then divided into *those with action capabilities* and those *engaged in deliberate action.* This distinction names the articulating concepts for the *self-care agency hierarchy* and *self-care hierarchy* respectively, bringing the "person" frame of reference into relationships with the subsumed "agency" and "action" frames of reference.

The selection of the most general concepts represented in the agency frame and in the action frame, namely, "self-care agency" as distinguished from "other forms of agency" (e.g., horticultural ability) and "self-care" as distinguished from "other forms of action" (e.g., gardening), is based on the presupposition that *action is for an end.* On this basis, the judgment was made that the deliberate actions of individuals as well as their capabilities for such actions are specialized according to types of end results sought. In thinking within an "agency frame" nurses focus on "self-care agency" as distinguished from "other forms of agency" and in the "action frame" on persons engaged in "self-care" as distinguished from their engagement in "other forms of action."

The *self-care agency hierarchy* is brought to closure in Figure 7-2 by the representation that "self-care agency" has distinct "elements" and each element has distinguishing "characteristics." The *self-care hierarchy* on the other hand can be made more specific by distinguishing distinct "systems of self-care" performed and still more specific through the identification of "discrete actions" within each system.

The concepts and relationships represented in Figure 7-2 suggest that nurses must be able to (1) think in three frames of reference — person, agency, and action, and (2) move their thinking from one frame of reference to each of the others as they work with individuals and groups. The organization of knowledge around each of the conceptual constructs named in Figure 7-2 and its mastery by nurses are essential for both effective nursing practice and research. The identification and organization of available, authoritative knowledge within the hierarchies of concepts is the proper work of nursing scholars.

Questions for Inquiry and Questions for Practice
The hierarchy of concepts represented in the "agency frame" in Figure 7-2 and their relationship to concepts represented

in the "action frame" and "person frame" suggest questions for inquiry. Such questions guide inquiry toward the further development of a body of knowledge about self-care agency. Three broad questions for inquiry are suggested.

1. What are the component parts (elements) of self-care agency and how are these parts related?
2. What are the distinguishing characteristics of each of the component parts of self-care agency and what is the range over which the characteristics of each part can vary?
3. What would constitute a sufficiency of evidence for asserting that
   a. the component elements of self-care agency are existent?
   b. the distinguishing characteristics of each component element of self-care agency are existent at specific values?

The work of answering these questions is the proper work of theorists, scholars, and researchers. Knowledge from other disciplines as well as newly formulated theories, hypotheses, laws, and bodies of factual information ensuing from inquiry that is guided by the formulated questions would constitute a body of theoretical knowledge descriptive and explanatory of "self-care agency." Such a body of knowledge would have its origin in a general theory of nursing (theoretically practical nursing science). It would constitute an *applied science,* since its constructs would include the relationships of concepts descriptive and explanatory of self-care agency with points of theory from other disciplines of knowledge, for example, psychology and human physiology. The development of an applied science of self-care agency is viewed as a necessary step in nursing's movement toward maturity as a profession.

There is also a need in nursing for a body of practical knowledge [9] to give guidance and direction to practitioners as they confront questions of nursing practice. Questions of practice include, for example: What at this time are the self-care capabilities of this person or these persons under nursing care? What can be projected about self-care capabilities for a future time period(s)? The questions of nursing practice that focus on self-care agency (capability for engagement in self-care) correlate with questions of inquiry previously enumerated. The formulation and expression of rules of practice as related to components and characteristics of self-care agency of persons under nursing care would constitute a section of a body of practical knowledge, a practical science [9], of self-care agency. Rules of practice would provide answers to the questions: What are valid and reliable means for the determination of the presence or absence of X component of self-care agency? Or, given the absence of X component of self-care agency in an individual, what means of helping are both valid and reliable?

Ideally, nurses would move in an organized manner toward the development of bodies of theoretical knowledge and related bodies of practical knowledge about self-care agency. The bodies of knowledge could be organized by types of nursing practice situations for individuals, families, and communities.

THE COMPONENTS OF SELF-CARE AGENCY

Inquiry to identify and describe the component parts of self-care agency can begin with an analysis of the expressed concept. Proceeding on this basis, the original NDCG definition of self-care agency, which expressed a formulated concept (p. 118), was analyzed to isolate (1) the broad conceptual elements within the concept (dominant themes), and (2) the expressed or implied relationship among the identified elements. Following this, the identified broad conceptual elements of the expressed concept were investigated to identify their substantive structure (i.e., the concepts that underlie them). The results are reported.

Broad Conceptual Elements

Three broad conceptual elements were isolated from the statement about self-care agency (p. 118). These include the following:

1. Power or capability to engage in two specified types of actions, that is,

2. The estimative operations of self-care, and
3. The productive operations of self-care

No one of the three elements can stand in isolation since the second and third elements, which specify types of action, make the first element a specific power. The term *operation* is used in the sense of process or action system. Estimative operations of individuals are action systems performed with a goal of determining what is to be done with respect to self-care while productive actions are performed with the goal of meeting existent and known self-care requirements with their regulatory orientations using particular technologies.

These broad conceptual elements are represented in Figure 7-3. The figure shows the elements in their relationships to each other and in relationship to individual human beings. The lines indicating relationship among the elements shown in the figure express that the element power (I) with its two qualifiers, estimative and productive operations (II and III), is a quality or characteristic that is integral to individuals. The power that is self-care agency is delimited not only by the two named types of operations but also by the relationship between the operations. This relationship is a two-way relationship since "estimative operations" precede "productive operations," but once productive operations are started there may be a need to perform further "estimative operations" (refer to p. 191 for a further development of the relationship).

This analysis of the NDCG's expressed concept of self-care agency to reveal its broad conceptual elements reflects in part the early insight of some NDCG members that *self-care agency* has the nature of an action (behavioral) repertoire (p. 118).

The Concepts Underlying Estimative and Productive Self-Care Operations
Explication of the substantive structure of self-care agency involved an investigation of each broad conceptual element (Fig. 7-3). The approach that was utilized first addressed the two types of operations and then the power or capability for

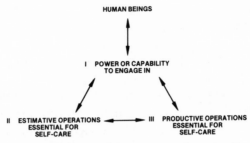

Figure 7-3   Three elements of the conceptual construct, self-care agency.

engaging in them. This approach was based on the assumption that:

1. The human power or capability that is named self-care agency is a power for engagement in specific types of action.
2. Two of the conceptual elements, estimative operations and productive operations for self-care, make the third element, the *human power* or *capability for such actions* a specific and not a general power.

The insight that self-care agency is a power for engagement in estimative and productive operations for self-care was grounded in the nature of practical endeavors, namely, that insights about and awareness of what is to be done precedes the doing [6, pp. 610—612]. Estimative and productive operations thus focus on two different but related types of action systems with different goal orientations.

In estimative type operations, the way of acting is that of *investigation or inquiry.* In *productive type operations* the way of acting is that of *regulation* (i.e., *bringing about change in* or *maintaining* some condition or state). The goal orientation of individuals who have capabilities for engaging in estimative type self-care operations is to acquire and use (1) empirical knowledge of self and environment that is adequate for making judgments about *what is,* and (2) technical knowledge of *what can be,* that is, whether existent conditions in self or environment can be regulated, to what degree, and by what regulatory measures. The goal orientation of individuals who have capabilities for productive type operations is to bring about the *regulation* (changing or maintaining) of existent conditions in themselves or the environment.

The movement from estimative to productive type operations is conceptualized as accomplished by two operations. One operation seeks to answer the question *what should be.* The goal orientation of persons with capabilities for this type of operation is to have knowledge of (1) the effects and results to be expected if regulatory action is taken or not taken; and (2) the similarities and differences expressed in terms of effects, results, and costs among possible courses of action open for choice for effecting regulations. This operation involves a discernment of the possibilities for and limits of change, or for the maintenance of some condition or state.

Individuals' hierarchies of values will afford the criterion measures that will guide the making of judgments about *what should be.* Such judgments are affirmations that one course of action or some combination of courses of action is to be preferred over other courses of action or that none should be pursued. Values within individuals' hierarchies of values — social, cultural, economic, health-oriented, religious, and spiritual — become operational as motivating forces. *A final affirming judgment* is about *what should be done ideally* with consideration of existing conditions, factors, and circumstances that will condition any regulation that is attempted. Making such judgments involves the use of both empirical and technical knowledge in reasoning.

The final transition from estimative to productive type operations is effected by individuals' decisions about *what will be done.* The decision as to what will be done may or may not be congruous with the judgment about *what should be done.* Harnett's basic psychologic model of action (Fig. 6-1) identifies, from a number of disciplines of knowledge, the *psychologic features of* and *the kinds of factors that can condition* the making of a decision about *what is to be done.* If *decision* is substituted for "Personal Action" in the model, the model serves to express many components of the process of decision making from a person perspective.

The substantive structure of the estimative and productive operations of self-care is summarized in the form of a charting of operations and results. Estimative, transitional, and productive operations with their results are identified in sequential order in time. Movement within and between the named operations should be understood.

SELF-CARE OPERATIONS AND RESULTS

Operations	Results
Estimative Type	
1. Investigation of internal and external conditions and factors significant for self-care	Empirical knowledge of self and environment
2. Investigation of the meaning of characterized conditions and factors and their regulation	Experiential knowing (based in part on acquired technical knowledge) of the meaning of the existent conditions and factors for life, health, and well-being
3. Investigation of the question: how can existent conditions and factors be regulated (i.e., changed or maintained)?	Technical knowledge of what can be regulated and the means available for effecting regulation
Transitional Type	
4. Reflection to determine which course of self-care should be followed	An affirming judgment that one course of self-care is preferred, or that a series of courses is preferred, or that none should be pursued
5. Deciding what to do with respect to self-care	A decision to engage in or not engage in specific regulatory self-care operations
Productive Type	
6. Preparation of self, materials, or environmental settings for the performance of a regulatory type self-care operation	Conditions of readiness for performing self-care operations for regulatory purposes
7a. Performance of productive self-care operations with specific regulatory purposes within a time period	Knowledge that regulatory measures are in process or are completed

7b. Determining presence of and monitoring, during performance, conditions known to affect effectiveness of performance and results

Information that conditions and factors affecting performance and results
a. Are or are not present
b. Are or are not under control if present

8. Monitoring for evidence of effects and results
   a. Desired
   b. Untoward

Information about events indicating that regulation is
a. Being achieved
b. Not being achieved
Knowledge of untoward results
a. Absence of
b. Presence of

9. Reflection to determine evidence of and adequacy of regulatory results

An affirming judgment as related to specific self-care regulatory operations
a. Self-care should continue
b. Self-care should be discontinued
   (1) To be resumed at a specific time
   (2) Not to be resumed as related to the operations in question

10a. Decision about regulatory operations
   a. Continue action
   b. Close action
   c. Cease action but resume at a specific time

10b. Decision about estimative operations
   a. Continue to use results obtained from estimative operations (current data base)
   b. Begin a new series of estimative operations

The Concepts Underlying the Power Element of Self-Care Agency

Following the exposition of the substantive structure of self-care operations, the power or capability element of self-care

agency was investigated. The investigative process was guided
by the following assumptions:

1. Self-care agency is a complex, acquired, human characteristic or
   quality.
2. Self-care agency when conceptualized as a human *power* is constituted from or associated with distinct capabilities that are empower-
   ing for engagement in estimative, transitional, and productive self-
   care operations and therefore have existence prior to an individual's
   engagement in these operations.

The idea of two structural levels, namely, the level of enabling
capabilities and the level of self-care operations, guided inquiry. The notion expressed in the second assumption, that
capabilities enabling for self-care operations would be first in
the order of existence, led to focusing inquiry on the question: What human capabilities must be existent (i.e., developed
and capable of being operationalized) before individuals can
engage in estimative, transitional, and productive self-care
operations? The response to the question was visualized as a
set of human capabilities that would be directly enabling for
estimative, transitional, and productive self-care operations
and without which these operations could not be performed.

The described *estimative self-care operations* are operations
of inquiry and as such seek both empirical knowledge and
technical knowledge for the purposes of understanding what
is and what can be brought about within a self-care frame of
reference. The *transitional operation of judging* what should
be done with respect to self-care is grounded in an individual's
knowledge, experience, and values and in the individual's
understanding of the situation of action. The *transitional
operation of deciding* what is to be done brings the individual
into confrontation with what the individual *knows about
self-care* as this relates to what the individual *values* and what
the individual *will do.* Finally, *productive operations* are
making and doing operations: preparing for regulatory operations; performing regulatory operations; monitoring regulatory operations and their effects and results; judging results
achieved; and deciding to continue or not to continue the

regulatory operations of self-care. These types of operations require the use of empirical and theoretical knowledge, the exercise of a range of skills, as well as sensorimotor functioning.

With these characteristics of self-care operations in mind, it was concluded that human capabilities (i.e., the human power for self-care operations) would be of a nature intermediate between (1) human functions physiologically or psychologically identified and named (e.g., sensation, memory, reasoning), and (2) the named types of self-care operations or processes and their results. Components of the power element would thus articulate with one or some combination of the estimative, transitional, and productive self-care operations.

The process of formulating and expressing the power components of self-care agency was facilitated by insights acquired prior to engagement in inquiry to identify the substantive structure of self-care agency. Some of these insights are reported in Chapter 8. Ten components of the power element of self-care agency were formulated and are expressed as follows:

Power Components of Self-Care Agency

1. Ability to maintain attention and exercise requisite vigilance with respect to (a) self as self-care agent and (b) internal and external conditions and factors significant for self-care
2. Controlled use of available physical energy that is sufficient for the initiation and continuation of self-care operations
3. Ability to control the position of the body and its parts in the execution of the movements required for the initiation and completion of self-care operations
4. Ability to reason within a self-care frame of reference
5. Motivation (i.e., goal orientations for self-care that are in accord with its characteristics and its meaning for life, health, and well-being)
6. Ability to make decisions about care of self and to operationalize these decisions
7. Ability to acquire technical knowledge about self-care from authoritative sources, to retain it and operationalize it
8. A repertoire of cognitive, perceptual, manipulative, communication, and interpersonal skills adapted to the performance of self-care operations

9. Ability to order discrete self-care actions or action systems into relationships with prior and subsequent actions toward the final achievement of regulatory goals of self-care
10. Ability to consistently perform self-care operations, integrating them with relevant aspects of personal, family, and community living

The mode for formalizing and expressing capabilities was selected in the interest of accuracy and conciseness of thought and economy of expression. Capabilities were expressed as a single series and not in categories for estimative, transitional, and productive type self-care operations.

The association of the ten named *power components* of self-care agency with self-care operations identified on pages 192–193 were explored. The conclusion was reached that all but one of the ten named power components usually would be associated with each of the ten identified self-care operations. The "ability to control the position of the body and its parts . . ." was identified as *not necessarily* associated with the "transitional operations" of making judgments and decisions about self-care or with the "productive operations" of reflection (Item 9) and decision (Items 10a and 10b).

The position is taken that the associations between some power components of self-care agency and some self-care operations are more significant than associations between others (Table 7-1). For example, "attention and requisite vigilance . . .", while necessary for all operations, are critical for operations to acquire empirical and technical knowledge (operations 1, 2, 3, and 8). This power also is critical for operations 6 and 7 in periods of skill development and effective habit formation. Power component "ability to make decisions about care of self and to operationalize such decision" is viewed as associated with each one of the named self-care operations (since all operations contain decision-making elements) but as critical for transitional operation "deciding what to do with respect to self-care."

The ten capabilities identified as constituting the *power element* of the concept self-care agency are considered as formulations in need of review and testing. Their value rests in their identification of a level of human capabilities that

Table 7-1   Associations Among the Power and Operations Components of Self-Care Agency

| | Substantive Components of Self-Care Agency | | |
| | Self-Care Operations Components | | |
Power Components[a]	Estimative[b]	Transitional[b]	Productive[b]
1. Maintaining attention and requisite vigilance	1, 2, 3	4, 5	6, 7, 8, 9, 10
2. Controlled use of available physical energy	1, 2, 3	4, 5	6, 7, 8, 9, 10
3. Control of the position of the body and its parts in execution of movements	1, 2, 3		6, 7, 8
4. Reasoning within a self-care frame of reference	1, 2, 3	4, 5	6, 7, 8, 9, 10
5. Motivations or goal orientation to self-care	1, 2, 3	4, 5	6, 7, 8, 9, 10
6. Decision-making about self-care	1, 2, 3	4, 5	6, 7, 8, 9, 10
7. Acquiring, retaining and operationalizing technical knowledge about self-care	1, 2, 3	4, 5	6, 7, 8, 9, 10
8. Having a repertoire of skills for self-care	1, 2, 3	4, 5	6, 7, 8, 9, 10
9. Ordering discrete self-care actions	1, 2, 3	4, 5	6, 7, 8, 9, 10
10. Integrating self-care operations with other aspects of living	1, 2, 3	4, 5	6, 7, 8, 9, 10

[a]See pages 195–196 for full expressions of the components.
[b]Numbers correspond with those on pages 192–193.

occupies an intermediate position between self-care operations and physiologically or psychologically described capacities of human beings. From a structuring of knowledge perspective, the identified capabilities serve as essential links for the articulation of knowledge from a number of disciplines of knowledge with the concept self-care agency.

If the ten named power components of self-care agency have their foundations in natural or acquired aspects of human functioning, it can be assumed that self-care agency varies with the time-specific values of each of the ten components and with the relationships among the ten components. This assumption raises a number of questions for inquiry, including the following:

1. What are the range and the limits of the range over which each power component can vary?
2. Within which segment(s) of the range over which a power component can vary is the value of the component sufficient for engagement in specific self-care operations?
3. What meaning does the absence of a sufficient degree of each power component have for an individual?
4. What are the possibilities for power components existent at one degree for movement to other degrees?
5. What factors are associated with the movements of power components from one degree to other degrees?
6. What are possible patterns of coexistence in individuals of the ten power components?
7. What is the human and the nursing meaning of each identified pattern of coexistence of the ten power components of self-care agency?
8. What means are available for effective changes in the degree (value) of each power component or in maintaining the component at a specific degree?

The significance of these questions for nursing practice is self-evident. Nurses engaged in practice are in strategic positions to study the power components of self-care agency as they reveal themselves in individuals under nursing care. The eight formulated questions can guide inquiry by giving direction to the kinds of data to be collected and to its organization. Scholars and researchers can make major contributions to the development of a science of self-care agency by examining the nursing legitimacy of the eight questions and by affording them appropriate priority positions in their endeavors.

The foregoing exposition of the substantive structure of the *power* element of self-care agency is viewed by the NDCG as contributing to the development of an essential segment of a body of knowledge descriptive of and explanatory of self-care agency. In the investigation of the conceptual element, power to engage in self-care operations, the hypothetico-deductive approach was used *to move* from (1) insights about practical endeavors and (2) ten described self-care operations *to* identification of and judgments about the power components of self-care agency. The compositive (gathering together) mode for development of this knowledge explanatory of self-care agency is evident [9, p. 313].

SUMMARY

The work of analysis of the broad conceptual structure of self-care agency and the identification of the substantive structure of each of three initially identified broad conceptual elements have produced new theoretical formulations about self-care agency. Starting with a general concept of self-care agency, two substantive conceptual structures were identified.

One construct rests on the assumption that there are ten distinct kinds of self-care operations grouped in three categories and that these operations are related in a time sequence of before and after and that all operations are essential for self-care.

The second structure is grounded in the assumption that the power that is self-care agency is constituted from ten distinct power components each of which is associated with all or some self-care operations. No associations among the power components were posited. That there are probable associations is recognized.

The relationship between the two constructs can be formulated as a "factor relating theory" [10]. In such a form it can facilitate movement toward continuing development of a body of descriptive and explanatory knowledge about self-care agency.

Figure 7-2 can help to identify that the inquiry reported here and the questions for inquiry that were formulated focus on "elements of self-care agency" within the *Agency Frame*. Work with the two expressed conceptual constructs by nurse practitioners, scholars, and researchers should contribute to the advancement of knowledge of "elements of self-care agency" including "characteristics of elements" (i.e., how the power elements and the self-care operation elements are revealed in the real world of the nurse).

REFERENCES

1. Parsons, T. *The Structure of Social Action,* Vol. I. New York: Macmillan Free Press Paperback, 1968.
2. Parsons, T., and Shils, E. A. (Eds.). *Toward a General Theory of Action.* New York: Harper & Row, 1951.
3. Kotarbinski, T. *Praxiology* (translated by O. Wojtasiewicz). New York: Pergamon, 1966.
4. Macmurray, J. *Self as Agent.* London: Faber & Faber, 1966.
5. Barnard, C. I. *The Functions of the Executive.* Cambridge, Mass.: Harvard University Press, 1938. Pp. 200–211.
6. Lonergan, B. J. F. *Insight.* New York: Philosophical Library, 1958. Pp. 3–14.
7. Nursing Development Conference Group. Minutes of the Meeting of Nov. 1, 1969 (typewritten).
8. Phenix, P. H. *Realms of Meaning.* New York: McGraw-Hill, 1964. Pp. 324–326.
9. Maritain, J. *The Degrees of Knowledge.* New York: Scribner's, 1959. Pp. 311–316, 459.
10. Dickoff, J., James, P., and Wiedenback, E. Theory in a practice discipline. *Nurs. Res.* 17:421, 1968.

Self-Care Agency: Diagnostic Considerations

DIAGNOSIS: A FUNCTION OF NURSES
It is the function of nurses to be concerned with the immediate as well as the future well-being of patients. Caring for individuals or groups from this perspective is an essential dimension of the professional form of nursing practice. This form of practice involves nurses in diagnostic-type endeavors, in determinations of what can and should be done, and in the selection and use of appropriate methods of helping for the achievement of regulatory results through self-care or through the regulation of self-care agency. Diagnosis precedes other nursing endeavors, since through it the conditions and factors existent in individuals and groups that have significance for self-care and nursing are identified.

Diagnosis is for the purpose of enabling nurses to know and to focus on existent conditions that are associated with self-care requirements and self-care agency of persons or groups under their care. Nurses' actions performed with the goal of making an accurate diagnosis, for example, of self-care agency of an individual or of all the members of a family, are a form of nursing care. Nurses who use the conceptual construct "nursing process" relate diagnosis to the *assessment phase* of the process.

Diagnostic actions of nurses are oriented to the question: *What is?* Results of diagnostic endeavors have the form of empirical knowledge of *what is* and *what is in process* in a person or a group under nursing care. This knowledge, ideally, is communicated by nurses to the person or group under nursing care in a prudent and comprehensible manner [1]. Subsequently, it is the *meaning* that nurse and patient attach to the *characterizing judgments* about *what is* that motivates a nurse to investigate and make judgments about *what can and should be done* with respect to *self-care* and *self-care*

201

agency. Ideally, it is the person or group under nursing care who decides *what will be done* when the reality and the technically based options for regulation (according to the best judgment of the nurse(s)) are made clear. When person(s) under nursing care are incapable of making decisions about their own self-care or the protection or development of their self-care agency, nurses should involve in a significant way parents, guardians, or related adults in decision-making about the type of regulatory nursing[1] to be provided.

The professional approach to nursing practice as described here may not be commonly encountered in places where individuals or groups go for health care including nursing. A not infrequent approach of nurses and others is to fit an individual or group into an established routine [2], which may or may not be congruent with the condition of the individual or group seeking or in need of nursing.

Diagnosis in nursing seeks to achieve a number of goals. Ideally, diagnosis should be viewed as a patient-focused investigatory operation or series of operations (processes) to determine:

1. The human and environmental conditions and factors that are giving rise to requirements for self-care
2. The self-care that is being provided or has been provided
3. The evidence that existent self-care requirements are or are not being met
4. The internal and external conditions and factors that are interfering with meeting existent self-care requirements or in some way affect how they can be met
5. The qualitative and quantitative characteristics of self-care agency
6. Human states and internal and external factors that are conditioning the character, operability, or further development of self-care agency

Ideally, nursing diagnostic systems, like all diagnostic systems, should be dynamic, developmental, and etiologic. This

---

[1] Regulatory type nursing refers to nursing actions directed (1) to meeting self-care requirements of a person or group, and (2) to the effective protection, use, or development of self-care agency on the part of a person or members of a group. Nursing actions with regulatory goals are preceded by actions with diagnostic goals, and both types are performed within interpersonal situations.

ideal requires nurses to engage in patient-focused inquiry *at this time, over a period of time,* and at times *over prolonged periods*; requires them to move from a position of having *no* or little *empirical knowledge about patient or environment* to having an *increased amount of empirical knowledge* that is *generative of new knowledge and of new questions for inquiry*; and finally moves a nurse to the desired position of having evidence sufficient for reasonable pronouncements relative to each of the six named points of inquiry [3]. This ideal of nursing diagnosis may not be achievable in practice but it should guide the diagnostic goals sought by nurses. The relationship of diagnostic to regulatory nursing process must be kept in mind [4].

The medical dictum that *diagnosis precedes treatment* supplies nurses with an essential rule of nursing practice. Paraphrased for nursing practice, the rule would be: Diagnosis precedes the designing of nursing systems to meet self-care requirements of individuals or groups or to regulate the exercise or development of self-care agency. The rule applies not only to systematic diagnostic processes but also to the multiple but isolated diagnostic (investigatory) actions that nurses perform prior to their decisions about the appropriateness and validity of specific regulatory actions during the actual provision of regulatory type nursing care.

Some work of NDCG members in process during the 1970s that contributes directly or indirectly to the development of insights and practices relative to nursing diagnosis is presented. The reported work and its results is organized around the patient variable *self-care agency*. The specific merit of the work is the contribution made to the fifth and sixth points of nursing inquiry (p. 202) concerning characteristics of self-care agency and the internal and external factors that condition the adequacy, operability, or development of self-care agency.

THREE SCALES FOR GRADING SELF-CARE AGENCY
Three scales for use as aids in formulating and expressing judgments about the self-care agency of persons under nursing

care have been used by NDCG members since the early 1970s. The scales are named the Developmental, the Operative, and the Adequacy Scales. The bases for their development and use are expressed in the following propositions:

1. Self-care agency is an acquired human characteristic the formation of which varies with age, genetic and constitutional factors, and developmental state.
2. Self-care agency may be developed but not operative at points in time.
3. Self-care agency may be developed and operative but not enabling by reason of its quality or magnitude for the performance of specific self-care operations essential at a point in time to the life, functioning, or well-being of individuals or groups.

The scales, which have been through a number of revisions, are presented in Figure 8-1. They have the form of three graduated series of units that express (1) degree of development, (2) degree of operability of self-care agency, and (3) adequacy in relation to a known therapeutic self-care demand. The units for measuring self-care agency expressed in the developmental and operative scales are quantitative in character; in combination they are a means for grossly describing how much self-care agency an individual has at a specific time and how much is in operation. The adequacy scale units express results of *assessment* of self-care agency using the known therapeutic self-care demand as the standard for assessment.

The scales are diagnostic tools in the sense that they indicate the points of view from which self-care agency of individuals can and should be examined and the kinds of nursing judgments that should be made. The scales have utility in the initial and early phases of providing nursing for specific patients, when judgments about self-care agency may need to be based on readily available information about overt states, conditions, and factors (e.g., age, level of awareness, immobility). The utility of the scales during and after completion of specific diagnostic processes rests in the scales' identification of the kinds of nursing judgments to be made and in

DEGREES OF DEVELOPMENT OF SELF-CARE AGENCY

______ Undeveloped

______ Developing

______ Developed but not stabilized
- ______ in need of redevelopment
- ______ in process of redevelopment

______ Developed and stabilized
- ______ in need of redevelopment
- ______ in process of redevelopment
- ______ redeveloped and stabilized

______ Developed but declining

A

OPERABILITY OF SELF-CARE AGENCY

______ Not operative

______ Partially operative

______ Fully operative

B

TYPES OF SELF-CARE OPERATIONS	SELF-CARE AGENCY: ADEQUATE FOR OPERATIONS	SELF-CARE AGENCY: NOT ADEQUATE FOR OPERATIONS
***I ESTIMATIVE OPERATIONS ASSOCIATED WITH:**		
†A Universal self-care requirements	______	______
†B Developmental self-care requirements	______	______
†C Health-deviation self-care requirements	______	______
***II TRANSITIONAL OPERATIONS ASSOCIATED WITH:**		
A Universal self-care requirements	______	______
B Developmental self-care requirements	______	______
C Health-deviation type requirements	______	______
***III PRODUCTIVE OPERATIONS ASSOCIATED WITH MEETING**		
A Universal self-care requirements	______	______
B Developmental self-care requirements	______	______
C Health-deviation of self-care requirements	______	______

*These operations are described in Chapter 7.

†Universal self-care requirements are regulatory requirements that are common to all human beings with requisite adjustments for age, sex, development state, et cetera; developmental and health-deviation requirements are names for types of regulations necessitated respectively by developmental and health deviation processes or the control of same.

C

Figure 8-1 Self-care agency. *A.* Developmental scale. *B.* Operability scale. *C.* Adequacy scale.

the notion of a three-dimensional grading of self-care agency. This three-dimensional grading is essential to (1) identification of the range and limits of a patient's role in self-care, (2) the defining of nursing goals as related to a patient's self-care agency, and (3) the selection of valid and appropriate methods of helping a patient in meeting specific self-care requirements and in the regulation or development of self-care agency.

The scale units in Figure 8-1 refer to the kinds of *broad characterizing value judgments* that can be made about self-care agency. Characterizing value judgments in nursing and generally in the field of health care should be followed by *appraising value judgments* that express the meaning of a characteristic for the person who has that characteristic [5]. For example, the characterizing judgment that an adult person's *self-care agency* is *not operative* means that this person can have no instrumental role in self-care, and without help from responsible others, the person's life, health, and well-being are endangered.

The *developmental scale* expressive of the degree of development of self-care agency has scale units that are based on the assumption that all human beings can be divided into classes of persons with undeveloped, developing, and developed self-care agency. State of growth and development, biologically, psychologically, and psychosocially explained, is accepted as specifying human conditions and factors that determine the range of values that self-care agency can have at developmental periods throughout the life span of individuals. State of growth and development itself is associated with chronologic age, genetic and constitutional factors, and the sex of the individual as well as with health state and external environmental conditions.

The *operative scale* is designed to be responsive to the following nursing practice questions. Given a specific degree of development of self-care agency, is self-care agency operative at this time? Can it be expected to remain operative? If not, why not? The operative scale units are based on the assumption that given a degree of development, self-care agency can be fully operative, partially operative, or not operative at points in time. State(s) of human functioning, physiologically, psychologically, or psychosocially explained, are accepted as specifying the human and environmental conditions and factors that are associated with levels of operability of self-care agency.

The use of the *adequacy scale* by nurses presumes that they have knowledge of (1) a patient's self-care requirements; (2) the means or technologies that can be effectively used to meet them; and (3) the program of discrete actions to be performed in self-care. The use of this scale by nurses also presumes that they have knowledge of the degree of development and operability of self-care agency and of the conditions and factors that affect both development and operability. Backscheider's work with adult ambulatory patients with diabetes mellitus demonstrates the approaches and the diagnostic endeavors needed for nurses to make judgments about self-care agency of adult patients [6].

A nurse's location of a patient on each scale provides nurses with specific guides for the identification of nursing goals and for the selection and use of specific regulatory measures and ways of helping. For example, nurses' judgments and decisions about adults with partially operative self-care agency due to ambulatory restrictions will vary with conditions and factors associated with the character of the restrictions. In this frame of reference, persons on medically prescribed bed rest and persons with immobilized lower extremities because of fractures need different types of regulatory nursing to achieve different health goals. However, the combinations of ways of helping used by nurses may be similar for the two types of patients.

It is a patient's conjoined placement on the three self-care agency scales that provides nurses with the empirical bases for designing valid and reliable systems of regulatory nursing for persons or groups under nursing care. The possibilities for conjoined placements of individuals on the three scales is shown in Table 8-1. The possibilities represented assume that (1) measurement of self-care agency on one scale is inde-

Table 8-1 Association of Location on the Developmental Scale with Necessary or Possible Location on the Operative and Adequacy Scales

Developmental Scale for Self-Care Agency	Operative Scale			Adequacy Scale	
	Fully Operative	Partially Operative	Not Operative	Adequate	Not Adequate
Undeveloped self-care agency	*	*	*	—	N
Developing self-care agency	P	P	P	—	N
Developed self-care agency					
Not stabilized	P	P	P	P	P
Stabilized	P	P	P	P	P
Declining	P	P	P	P	P

* Scale not relevant.

N = Necessary conjoined placement; P = Possible conjoined placement.

pendent of measurement on the other scales; and (2) there are necessary as well as possible relationships between the developmental, operative, and adequacy values of self-care agency.

The necessary relationships indicated in Table 8-1 are between degree of *development* and *adequacy* and degree of *operability* and *adequacy*. Undeveloped or *developing self-care* agency can be equated with self-care agency that is *not adequate;* the same relationship exists for self-care agency that is *not operative or partially operative.* On the other hand, self-care agency that is *developed* and *fully operative* may be *adequate* or *not adequate* when judged against *a formulated therapeutic self-care demand.*

Conjoined placements of individuals on the self-care agency scales define the *social dependency* of persons under health care on others for the meeting of their continuing requirement for self-care. Conjoined placements also indicate the character of the social dependency by specifying the broad reasons for the existence of social dependency, namely, developmental or functional states or the nature of the self-care requirements and the actions necessary for meeting them. A patient's location on the three scales also points to the kinds of nursing goals that can and should be formulated for the person with respect to the development or the protection of their powers of self-care agency.

The scales at this stage of development have limited utility for nurses in practice settings. They indicate the kinds of patient information required for making judgments about self-care agency along the dimensions indicated. Information would include the following:

1. Time since birth — chronologic age
2. Developmental state, biologically, psychologically, and psychosocially explained
3. Functional state, physiologically, psychologically, and psychosocially explained
4. Internal and external factors affecting human development and functioning

5. Current and historical information about self-care that is consistently performed or not performed by or for individuals
6. The current and the projected demand for self-care that is essential for life, health, or well-being

Nurses' use of empirical knowledge about patients' self-care agency demands theoretical knowledge if nurses are to acquire and attach significance to patient information descriptive or explanatory of self-care agency. The continuing development of the self-care agency scales (including refinement of the scale units) should add substantially to a body of knowledge about self-care agency. Insights of the NDCG members about this process are reported in subsequent sections of this chapter.

Human Capabilities and Dispositions for Self-Care

In an article prepared in 1971 and published in 1974 [6], Backscheider reported the utility of a three-pronged approach to nursing diagnosis in a nursing clinic for ambulatory adults with diabetes mellitus. The approach involves (1) inquiry to determine the regulatory goals to be achieved through self-care and the regulatory measures to be used; (2) a detailed analysis of the foregoing to determine the specific estimative and productive self-care operations that would need to be performed to achieve the regulatory goals using specific measures; and (3) inquiry to determine the ability of patients to perform the actions that are the component elements of self-care operations.

The determination of the goals of and the measures to be used in self-care and their analysis from an action perspective provides the nurse with information about a patient's *therapeutic self-care demand* or a segment thereof. Inquiry about *self-care agency* provides the nurse with information about patients' self-care abilities and limitations. For example, a constituent part of the therapeutic self-care demand of some persons with diabetes mellitus is the regulation of blood glucose level through insulin as well as diet. The technology of insulin therapy involves the injection of the regulatory product into the tissues and the testing of urine to determine the presence of sugar. Implicit in this is the *action demand* to "manipulate small objects," "syringe, medicine dropper." This action demand requires "manual dexterity" and involves *fine control of the position and movement of the fingers* in the exercise of *manipulative skills.*

The three-pronged approach to nursing diagnosis has demonstrated utility in the design and provision of nursing for ambulatory adults with chronic disease processes that give rise to continuing self-care requirements of the health deviation type. Regulatory goals of self-care, measures used in achieving them, and action demands can be generalized to some degree for populations. Such generalizations provide models of constituent parts of *therapeutic self-care demands* that are associated with events resultant from specific disease processes and therapies [6].

One critical consideration in the use of this practice approach is the ability of nurses to think within an *action frame of reference* when dealing with the patient variable, *therapeutic self-care demand,* and the ability to think within an *agency frame of reference* when dealing with the patient variable, *self-care agency* (see Fig. 7-2). Significant to the latter are the approaches that nurses take to diagnose patients' powers of self-care agency.

A SURVEY LIST
Backscheider describes in the 1974 article her use of a survey list of the types of human capabilities requisite for engagement in self-care. Backscheider uses the term *general capabilities* with reference to listings of "physical, mental, motivational, emotional, and orientational capabilities" essential for engagement in self-care.

Backscheider's initial list of general capabilities has been consistently used by Crews as a guide to the assessment of self-care agency of patients in three nursing clinics for adults and by other NDCG members in teaching. The survey list of general capabilities with modifications by Anger, Crews, and Orem is presented as Figure 8-2.

CAPABILITIES AND DISPOSITIONS

CONDITIONING FACTORS & STATES	SELECTED BASIC CAPABILITIES		KNOWING AND DOING CAPABILITIES	DISPOSITIONS AFFECTING GOALS SOUGHT	SIGNIFICANT ORIENTATIVE CAPABILITIES & DISPOSITIONS
	I	II			
GENETIC & CONSTITUTIONAL FACTORS	SENSATION PROPRIOCEPTION EXTEROCEPTION	ATTENTION	RATIONAL AGENCY	SELF-UNDERSTANDING SELF-AWARENESS	ORIENTATIONS TO: TIME HEALTH OTHER PERSONS EVENTS, OBJECTS
AROUSAL STATE	LEARNING	PERCEPTION	OPERATIONAL KNOWING	SELF-IMAGE SELF-VALUE	PRIORITY SYSTEM OR VALUE HIERARCHY MORAL ECONOMIC AESTHETIC MATERIAL SOCIAL
SOCIAL ORGANIZATION	EXERCISE OR WORK	MEMORY	LEARNED SKILLS READING COUNTING WRITING VERBAL PERCEPTUAL MANUAL REASONING	SELF-ACCEPTANCE SELF-CONCERN ACCEPTANCE OF BODILY FUNCTIONS WILLINGNESS TO MEET NEEDS OF SELF	INTEREST & CONCERNS HABITS ABILITY TO WORK WITH THE BODY & ITS PARTS
CULTURE		CENTRAL REGULATION OF MOTIVATIONAL-EMOTIONAL PROCESSES			
EXPERIENCE	REGULATION OF THE POSITION & MOVEMENT OF THE BODY & ITS PARTS		SELF-CONSISTENCY IN KNOWING & DOING	FUTURE DIRECTEDNESS	ABILITY TO MANAGE SELF & PERSONAL AFFAIRS

Figure 8-2 A survey list of human capabilities and dispositions foundational to the human power, self-care agency, with a list of factors and states that condition the capabilities and dispositions.

212

The final revision of the survey list adheres to Backscheider's original design. There are naming changes for some items, some reordering of items, and introduction of additional items.

The revised survey list of "human capabilities and dispositions" is composed of five sections.

1. Selected Basic Capabilities I
2. Selected Basic Capabilities II
3. Knowing and Doing Capabilities
4. Dispositions Affecting Goals Sought [7]
5. Significant Orientational Capabilities and Dispositions

Each section is viewed as reflecting a conceptualized level of human capabilities and dispositions from an action perspective. For example, the sections, Selected Basic Capabilities I and II, identify human capabilities that are foundational to capabilities and dispositions identified in sections 3, 4, and 5. The entries within each of the five sections are viewed as interrelated in one or more combinations. The interrelationships among the sections can be examined from a psychophysiologic, a psychologic, or a psychosocial frame of reference.

In the final revision of the survey list, included items meet three criteria. The first criterion is that the items included in the list name unique human capabilities or dispositions as distinguished from more comprehensive states of individuals. For example, level of awareness as associated with arousal state was excluded from the section named Basic Capabilities II because of the "state" character of arousal and the knowledge that "attention" (the capability) is functional only within certain levels of arousal [8, 9] — the conclusion being that *attention* is the capability essential for *deliberate action* while "arousal state" *conditions attention* directed to this or to that.

The second criterion is that the items included in the list represent sets of human capabilities and dispositions that can be associated with one or more of the *ten abilities* that are hypothesized to constitute the *power element of self-care agency* (Chap. 7, pp. 195 and 196). Here the consideration is that particular values of combinations of the named *capabilities or dispositions* will be associated not only with some level of development or operability of the human abilities that together constitute the power element of self-care agency but also with the development and operability of other human abilities. Thus the named capabilities and dispositions are associated with self-care agency but also with other specific forms of human agency.

The third criterion is that each capability or disposition named in the survey list can be examined and explained (to some degree) in isolation from other capabilities or dispositions. For example, while attention, sensation, and memory are functionally inseparable, within frames of reference provided by physiology and psychology each one can be subjected to investigation to determine the value at which it is operational in an individual.

The survey list of human capabilities and dispositions is a construct in the nature of a beginning articulation of "points of theory" and "structures" from a number of disciplines of knowledge with the theoretical construct, self-care agency. Relating identified capabilities and dispositions to the ten hypothesized abilities that constitute the power element of self-care agency should lead to further insights about an applied science of self-care agency. This is one suggested approach to the further development of a body of knowledge about self-care agency meaningful for nursing diagnosis.

Another approach to the further development of such a body of knowledge (also meaningful for nursing diagnosis) is the specification of the kinds of information that can be sought about each capability or disposition. The following are examples of kinds of information to be sought in assessing the capacity of an individual for exercise or work. (Self-care is work.)

1a. Chemical energy in food intake available for transformation as heat or work

1b. Availability of oxygen for transformation of chemical energy in
the food intake
Efficiency of respiratory and circulatory adaptations during
exercise and work for oxygen absorption, transportation, and use
2a. Strength of musculature
2b. Sustaining of effort
2c. Accuracy and sureness of movement
3a. Fatigue from muscular activity
3b. Fatigue from activity of nervous system

In working with the named human capabilities and dispositions, their essentiality in the diagnosis of self-care agency
becomes clear since the capabilities and dispositions specify
the human foundations for the po∴er element of self-care
agency. From a diagnostic perspective they are *etiologic* in
relation to the qualitative and quantitative characteristics of
the self-care agency of individuals at points in time.

In the initial survey list (1971) Backscheider included four
types of factors that condition the identified general human
capabilities; namely, genetic and constitutional factors, social
organization, culture, and experience. These are included in
the final revision of the survey list (Fig. 8-2). A fifth factor
was added, namely, "arousal level." The relating of these
types of factors and states to the specific capabilities and
dispositions and to the development and operability of self-
care agency is a task to be done. For example, in clinical
practice Backscheider [10] identified "high stress, high-demand households" (a social organization factor) as a potentially detrimental type environment for the exercise or development of self-care agency by members of an adult,
ambulatory clinic population. In this example, a social organization factor has a potential for conditioning the capacity
for "exercise or work" (including self-care) as well as "Dispositions Affecting Goals Sought" and "Significant Orientational Capabilities and Dispositions" (Fig. 8-2).

CAPABILITIES AND DISPOSITIONS AND THE DESIGN OF NURSING SYSTEMS
In working with members of an adult, ambulatory population of a diabetic nurse management clinic, Backscheider

identified *major determiners* of the types and amounts of nursing assistance required by them [10]. Backscheider's *major determiners* were identified as one or some combination of the Human Capabilities and Dispositions and the Types of Conditioning Factors named in Figure 8-2.

The four most frequently noted determiners of the type and amount of nursing were identified as (1) operative knowing capabilities, (2) motivational-emotional dispositions, (3) capabilities for consistency of action and self-discipline associated with the conditioning factor Social Organization, and (4) a combination of *health orientation* with *time* and *priority orientations*. Low values of these human capabilities and dispositions resulted in high requirements for nursing with the nurse utilizing specialized modes of helping.

Backscheider's summarizations of the most frequently occurring determiners include reference to Orem's descriptions of *methods of assisting or helping* and types of nursing systems with their *role specifications for nurse and patient*. The notion of "determiners of nursing assistance" according to Backscheider is grounded in the following assumption expressed by Orem:

The condition which validates the existence of a requirement for nursing in an adult is *the absence of the ability to maintain for . . . self continuously that amount and quality of self-care which is therapeutic in sustaining life and health, in recovering from disease or injury, or in coping with their effects* [11].

The following summarizations were made by Backscheider:

Deficit in *operative knowing* is one of the major determiners of type and amount of nursing assistance within a clinic setting. Patients who can respond to only one factor, to only one factor at a time, or who can construct a system only on the basis of concrete factors are permanently limited in certain [self-care] procedures, if their clinic performance reflects their actual capacity. *Compensatory actions* to achieve the level of performance needed by the [self-care] regimen will have to come from the nurse herself or from a family member who has the capacity. Evidence that the patient has the required capacities but is not utilizing them in relation to his health state and its management is the justification for an *educative nursing system.*

Motivational-emotional deficits may arise from a number of sources; one being the type of household the patient comes from. High-stress, high-demand households and situations with limited emotional input are two potentially detrimental types of environments. The limitation which may arise from the first is the amount of available energy the patient is free to direct to himself. In this situation the important factor is his position in the household in relation to the management of the crisis. In situations with limited emotional input to the patient, the deficit is in the area of reinforcement to the patient of his own value and support in maintaining consistency in the regimen. *Compensatory actions* might range from recommending change in [the] environment to establishing an on-going system of *supportive nursing to the individual* and of *teaching and or support to the family.*

Deficits in consistency and self-discipline are another limitation which is a major determiner of the nature and extent of the nursing system. Evidence of potential for development in these areas would indicate the establishment of a strong *supportive-educative system.* Lack of such evidence would result in establishment of *minimal safe standards as the optimal level* [of performance] *expected of the patient* and of a system of *supportive-repetitive educational nursing care* to maintain the patient at that level.

Finally, *major deficits in health orientation* combined with *lack of time and priority orientation* probably signal unsatisfactory patient performance, especially when this state results from the cultural environment and when the patient is dependent on orientation to that environment. *Educative measures directed to the patient's significant others and an extensive educative-supportive system directed to the patient* may be indicated when there is evidence of capacity and willingness to change. In this case, effort must be made to examine in detail the on-going living pattern and to help patient and family structure in the desired system of care [10, italics added].

The four major determiners of type and amount of required nursing assistance identified by Backscheider in an adult clinic population could, all things being equal, be tentatively predicted as existent in populations of ambulatory adults comparable with respect to age, sex, and experiential backgrounds. The determiners would not hold true for nonambulatory acutely ill populations.

Backscheider's work of identifying *major determiners of requirements* of members of a clinic population *for nursing* is an indicator of the meaning that *nursing diagnosis of self-care agency* has for the design and delivery of nursing care. It also is an indicator that the *Survey List of Human Capabilities and Dispositions Associated with Self-Care Agency* provides the structures for nurses' organization of behavioral data resulting from their observations of patients from which nurses can make inferences about the self-care abilities and limitations of persons under care.

A FURTHER DEVELOPMENT OF THE SURVEY LIST

The development of subcategories for the human capabilities and dispositions identified in the survey list is an essential step if the survey list is to become a practical tool for use in the diagnosis of self-care agency. The development of subcategories could accomplish two ends: (1) the identification of the range over which each capability and disposition could vary, and (2) the identification of the range over which the capabilities and dispositions do vary for specific nursing populations.

Backscheider's work toward the development of subcategories for the capability "structure of intellectual operations" or modes of operational knowing (Knowing and Doing Capabilities, Fig. 8-2) is reported in the next section. Her work was focused on an adult, ambulatory nursing clinic population. Some persons comprising the population had not had the benefits derived from formal education and could not read or write. Data about modes of operational knowing obtained from the nursing clinic population yielded three subcategories identified as follows:

A. Intellectual operations are experientially oriented and here-and-now focused.
B. Intellectual operations are oriented to concrete and experiential wholes with some understanding of their parts and boundaries.
C. Intellectual operations involve knowing within logical frameworks.

The subsequent section explains the process of identifying subcategories A and B for the capability *operational knowing*.

Knowing Capabilities in an Adult Population

It is with a high degree of respect that the NDCG presents a summary of Joan Backscheider's work in diagnosing self-care agency along the dimension of the human capability of operational knowing or thinking. The population was comprised of ambulatory adults. The setting for the investigation was a diabetic nurse management clinic within a medical center.

The frame of reference that guided the operations of the clinic was that of nursing system (see p. 107). Knowledge from medical and nursing sources about individuals with diabetes mellitus provided the basis for structuring a curriculum for use with members of the clinic population who were confronted with demands for acquiring new knowledge and skills for self-care. Individualized nursing assessment was a part of clinic operation. Questions of concern to a nurse in such a clinic in making an assessment include the following:

1. In what self-care does this person now engage? Are adjustments needed? If so, why?
2. What are the presenting requirements for regulation of the diabetic condition? What factors are conditioning the value of each of these requirements?
3. What means are available for meeting these regulatory requirements? What factors are conditioning the selection or the use of means or measures for meeting presenting requirements?
4. What self-care operations must be performed effectively and consistently to meet these regulatory requirements using specified means?
5. What self-care abilities are needed to engage in these self-care operations?

It was identified that the majority of persons comprising the clinic population functioned within either *partly compensatory* or *supportive developmental* nursing systems [10]. In both nursing systems, one essential method of helping utilized by the nurse was teaching toward the goal of knowledge and skill development. Both individual and group instructional sessions were conducted. During the initial period of clinic operation there was evidence that some persons did not acquire or did not use new knowledge toward the goal of regulating their diabetic condition.

In the role of nonparticipant observer of the instructional sessions, Backscheider made behavioral observations of the exchanges between the nurse and the patients noting the features of the patients' verbalizations. Backscheider was struck with the apparent conformity between patients' verbalizations and Piaget's and Furth's findings about how individuals think about objective reality [12].

At a previous time and for a different purpose Backscheider had studied and subsequently charted in table form the expressed inferences of Piaget, Furth, and Bruner [13] about the structure of intellectual operations of individuals according to the developmental periods and levels elaborated in Piaget's theory of the stage development of intelligence.

Backscheider used as a frame of reference from these sources *five levels of thinking* and *eight ranges or schemas of intellectual operations* (i.e., "operations of thought"). The levels of thinking are (1) sensorimotor; (2) preoperational; (3) concrete operational; (4) formal operational, low level; and (5) formal operational, high level. The eight ranges or schemas of intellectual operations were

1. Range of operative knowing
2. Range of conceptualization
3. Range of abstraction
4. Scheme of classification
5. Scheme of probability
6. Range of symbolization
7. Scheme of relating
8. Scheme of ordering

The "table of states" used by Backscheider thus was constituted of *forty cells* that associated eight ranges or schemas of *intellectual operations* with five *levels of thinking*. The "table of states" served in expressing judgments and inferences based on the verbalizations of patients expressive of their thinking about diabetes mellitus and their use of knowledge in caring for themselves as diabetic.

Observations were made during live and recorded interchanges between patients and the nurse. Backscheider's task was tridimensional. It involved (1) making observations of verbal exchanges in an interpersonal setting; (2) making inferences about the structure of the intellectual operations of patients on the basis of the behavioral data, verbal exchange data; and (3) classification of patients' expressions of what they knew and did in relation to their inferred intellectual operations.

Backscheider's ultimate goal was the development of a classification system valid for an adult clinic population along the dimension of the human capability of operational knowing or thinking. Such a classification system is viewed as essential for the type of nursing diagnosis of self-care agency that is dynamic, developmental, and etiologic. It is essential also whenever the deficit for engagement in effectively regulatory self-care is due to an absence or an insufficiency of knowledge or skills and whenever valid modes of helping are instructional and developmental in nature.

Some of Backscheider's expressed findings and conclusions from the exploratory investigation of operational thinking in an adult ambulatory population are reported. The manner of reporting findings reflects the complex process of data collection and inference-making as well as the analysis and synthesis of findings.

Two Groups of Patients
The most general conclusion reached was that in the adult, ambulatory population of one diabetic nurse management clinic there were some persons whose inferred operations of thought did not conform to those associated with the "formal operational level" (i.e., reasoning on "propositional verbal statements"). It was further concluded that these persons could be divided into two groups, namely, persons whose *inferred operations of thought* conformed either to "preoperational thinking" or "concrete operational thinking" as described by Piaget. For purposes of this report, these groups will be referred to as Group A and Group B, respectively. Persons in Group A were characterized by mental operations that were primarily experience-oriented with a

focus on the here and now, while persons in Group B were characterized by mental operations that were focused on concrete or experienced wholes with some understanding of relationships and boundaries. Backscheider formulated and expressed six "descriptors" of the mental operations for subcategories A and B of the clinic population [14]. The descriptors are presented along with observational information in Figures 8-3 and 8-4.

The practical significance of Backscheider's behavioral observations leading to formulation and expression of distinguishing characteristics of an adult clinic population rests not only in the resulting subcategories for the existent situations of operational knowing but also in the meaning that the subcategories have for the nurses' selection of valid ways of helping persons so characterized. For the subcategories to have meaning for the selection of valid ways for helping individuals in their meeting of demands for regulatory self-care, nurses must have understanding of how individuals' mental operations affect (1) new learning, and (2) what individuals can do at any point in time with respect to self-care because of their modes of thinking.

Intellectual Operations in a Clinic Population
On the basis of the observational data and the characterizing judgments made about clinic patients along the capability of operational knowing, Backscheider made and expressed inferences about the mental operations of persons observed. Inferences were expressed for seven types of intellectual operations of persons in Groups A and B. These operations are:

1. Concept formation
2. Symbol formation
3. Classifying
4. Using experience to arrive at a concept or to categorize
5. Relating events
6. Viewing self in relation to a situation
7. Predicting outcomes

Guidelines for Characterizing Individuals by their Intellectual Operations, Group A

GROUP A — Experientially oriented mental operations, here-and-now focused.

Characteristic 1. Expressed generalizations extend only to concrete personal experiences (involving self or others).

Examples: Diabetes is "sugar in your blood"
"sugar in your urine"
"losing your legs"

Starch is "potatoes"
"bread"
"rice"

Insulin is "a medicine"

Characteristic 2. Expectations of what or how things might occur take into account only what has already happened. They might take into account that more of the same might occur.

QUESTIONS	RESPONSES
What happens when your blood sugar is high?	"I don't know; it has never happened to me."
How do you feel when your blood sugar is low?	"Weak and shaky" (all other possible symptoms denied on the basis that they have never happened).

Characteristic 3. Learning about an unexperienced or a future event is most successful when it is followed by an experience with that event.

INSTRUCTION	SEQUENCE OF EVENTS
Sugar in the urine will show up as one of these colors (colors shown).	1) Demonstration → 2) occurrence of color change → 3) learning color as a symbol for sugar.
Peak time for insulin activity will come X hours after you take it.	1) Insulin is taken without an adequate food intake several weeks after the instruction is given; 2) the effects and results of this are not related to insulin activity.

Figure 8-3   Six characteristics of a subgroup of a nursing clinic population, Group A. (Courtesy of Joan E. Backsheider, R.N., Ph.D.)

Characteristic 4. Does not distinguish appropriate, prescribed means for goal achievement from nonappropriate, personally selected means.

Personal Experience Recounted	*Nurse Identified Problems*
"I bathe and oil my skin every day but the sore is getting worse."	Uses an unprescribed, strong, medicated ointment.
"I eat the amount of bread just like the dietitian said and I am still running 4+."	Is substituting cake or dressing for bread.

Characteristic 5. Can perform specific tasks effectively but cannot create order without explicit directives.

TASKS IN SEQUENCE	*REQUIREMENT*
1. Check urine in morning. 2. Take medication. 3. Eat.	Needs explicit list for organization of the tasks, e.g. a) voiding first urine; b) collect and test second urine; c) take medicine, spelling out each step of administration if on insulin; d) eating.
3a. Follow diet plan developed by the nutritionist.	Describe diet in terms of concrete food items rather than food exchanges.

Characteristic 6. Needs to be told most relationships between several factors and comprehends only that they are related.

INSTRUCTION	*LEARNING*
Diet, activity, and medication are related.	Learns as a memory item. Cannot apply to own life without help.
Diet, stress, and blood sugar are related.	May identify: "stress makes my urine orange"; "medicine keeps my urine blue."

Figure 8-3 (continued)

Guidelines for Characterizing Individuals by Their Intellectual Operations, Group B

GROUP B — Mental operations focused on concrete or experienced wholes with some understanding of boundaries and relationships among parts.

Characteristic 1. Generalizations are made about concrete or experienced wholes that take into account space and time.

QUESTIONS	*RESPONSES*
What does *peak* time for insulin activity mean?	"When insulin *acts the most* which might be a long time after you take it."
What is starch?	"One kind of *food* which *makes sugar*; and the amount it makes depends on which starch it is — on how much is in it."

Characteristic 2. Images in the individual's mind identify the continuity of an object over time and sometimes through different states.

Expressions
   "Starch looks like *bread or rice* or *something* to you but to the blood they become *sugar.*"

   "Results of the urine test might be different colors but they all tell you something about sugar in the blood."

Characteristic 3. Can identify that there is a relationship between concrete entities though the extent or totality of the relationship is not comprehended.

Expressions
   "I've noticed I feel better when I stick to my diet and keep somewhat active."

   "When I get stressed, I notice I'm weak."

Characteristic 4. Concepts can be reversed and returned to a different state.

Expression
   "My urine went from blue to orange but if I watch my diet most likely I can get it to go back to blue again."

Figure 8-4   Six characteristics of a subgroup of a nursing clinic population, Group B. (Courtesy of Joan E. Backsheider, R.N., Ph.D.)

Characteristic 5. Can distinguish between goal and means used to achieve it. Can make observations about own effect on the situation.

Expressions
"I have been trimming my calluses to keep my foot in good shape but I think I cut a little too far."

"I tried to stick close to my diet for a few days so I could eat a little more at a party but I don't think it worked too well for I ran 4+ for a day."

Characteristic 6. Can understand the idea foundational to a procedure and can engage in some organization of an approach to it.

Expression
"I usually start fixing breakfast between my first and second specimens so that when I do test my urine I'll be ready to take my medicine and eat."

Figure 8-4 (continued)

Backscheider's expressed inferences about mental operations with supporting data are reported for Groups A and B in Figures 8-5 and 8-6 [14, pp. 2—3, 5—6].

DIAGNOSIS OF SELF-CARE AGENCY: A SUMMARY
Nursing diagnosis that is specific to self-care agency is concerned with the identification of the qualitative and quantitative characteristics of self-care agency and with the determination of the states and factors that condition its characteristics, its operability, or its further development. As a variable in a nursing system, *self-care agency* has as its referent a person's *ability to do a specific kind of work* while the variable *therapeutic self-care demand* expresses the *kinds and amounts of work to be done.* Failure of nurses to recognize and to accept this relationship may be in part the cause of nursing's prolonged neglect of the human power, self-care agency.

INTELLECTUAL OPERATIONS
GROUP A

I CONCEPT FORMATION

    1. CONCRETE EXPERIENCE A ⟶ MEMORY
       (SURFACE LEVEL)
    2. CONCRETE EXPERIENCE $A^{1,2,3,n\ TIMES}$ ⟶ PERMANENT BUT CONCRETE CONCEPT
       (SURFACE LEVEL)

    EXAMPLES
    1. MOTHER, SISTER, FRIEND WITH DIABETES LOST LEGS ⟶ DIABETICS LOSE LEGS
    2. EXTRA ACTIVITY ⟶ SHAKINESS ⟶ WATCH ACTIVITY

II SYMBOL FORMATION

    AN ACTION OR AN EXPERIENCE (AT SURFACE LEVEL) + CONCRETE MANIFESTATION = A SYMBOL CONSISTING OF A CONCRETE ATTRIBUTE

    EXAMPLE
    DO URINE TEST + A COLOR RESULT = COLOR AS SYMBOL OF SOMETHING ABOUT SUGAR (WHAT IS UNCERTAIN)

III CLASSIFYING

    DIFFERENCE IN CONCRETE RESULTS = A DIFFERENCE IN STATE OF A THING AT SURFACE LEVEL

    EXAMPLE
    COLOR OF URINE TEST VARIES FROM BLUE TO ORANGE = BLUE . . . ORANGE MEANS DIFFERENT AMOUNTS OF SUGAR

IV USING EXPERIENCE TO ARRIVE AT CONCEPT OR CATEGORIZE

    REALITY
    EXPERIENCE A AND/OR EXPERIENCE B AND/OR EXPERIENCE C = X

    EXAMPLE
    SHAKINESS WITH/OR WEAKNESS WITH/OR RACING HEART = HYPOGLYCEMIA

    OPERATION AT THIS LEVEL
    EXPERIENCE A   AT TIME 1
    EXPERIENCE B   AT TIME 2   = ARE NOT RELATED OR ARE NOT HYPOGLYCEMIA
    EXPERIENCE A AND C AT TIME 3
    EXPERIENCE A   AT TIME 4
    EXPERIENCE C AND B AT TIME 5

V RELATING EVENTS

    REALITY
    CONCRETE EXPERIENCE $\subseteq$ * TOTALITY OF CONDITIONS = X POINT OR STATE $\subseteq$ SYSTEM OF GLUCOSE
               (SOME NONPERCEPTIBLE)   METABOLISM

    EXAMPLE
    SHAKINESS IS ONE OF A NUMBER OF CHANGES THAT OCCUR = HYPOGLYCEMIA WHICH IS ONE COMPONENT OF A TOTAL RANGE OF THE SYSTEM OF GLUCOSE METABOLISM

    OPERATION AT THIS LEVEL
    1. CONCRETE EXPERIENCE(S)   = POINT OR STATE
       CONFUSION + DROWSINESS   = TOO MUCH SUGAR IN THE BLOOD
    2. CONCRETE EXPERIENCE(S)   = A CHANGE IN POINT OR STATE
    "FEEL SHAKINESS AND FEEL RESTLESS" + "EAT HARD CANDY" = "DON'T FEEL THAT WAY ANY MORE"
    (INTUITIVE RELATIONSHIP; NO UNDERSTANDING OF REASON FOR THE EFFECT)

VI VIEWING SELF IN RELATION TO SITUATION

    REALITY
    1. EXPERIENCE OR STATE + PRESCRIBED RANGE OF X AND TECHNIQUE FOR REGULATING X = IDEAL OUTCOME
    2. EXPERIENCE + JUDGMENT ABOUT AND WAY OF CARRYING OUT PRESCRIBED REGULATORY TECHNIQUE = ACTUAL OUTCOME

    EXAMPLE
    PRESCRIPTION: EAT SOME HARD CANDY WHEN HYPOGLYCEMIC TO ARRIVE AT NORMAL STATE
    WHAT WAS DONE: EATS CANDY BARS OR CAKE WHEN HYPOGLYCEMIC AND ARRIVES AT ABNORMAL STATE

    OPERATION AT THIS LEVEL
    "I DID WHAT YOU TOLD ME AND I FELT TERRIBLE "
    DOES NOT RECOGNIZE DEVIATION FROM THE PRESCRIPTION AND EFFECT OF OWN ACTIONS AND JUDGMENTS

VII PREDICTING OUTCOMES

    EXISTS ONLY FOR GROSS SENSORIMOTOR TASKS

---

*THE SYMBOL $\subseteq$ MEANS A PROPER SUBSET OF

Figure 8-5 Expressed inferences about seven types of intellectual operations characterized as experientially oriented and here-and-now focused. (Courtesy of Joan E. Backscheider, R.N., Ph.D.)

INTELLECTUAL OPERATIONS
GROUP B

I CONCEPT FORMATION

1. RECENT OR CURRENT CONCRETE EXPERIENCE A HAS $\quad \Bigg[$ TYPE (A) SURFACE LEVEL CHARACTERISTICS
   TYPE (B) LESS OVERT EMPIRICAL CHARACTERISTICS

2. CONCRETE EXPERIENCE A $^{1,2,3n\ TIMES}$ + EXPERIENCING OF OCCURRENCE OF TYPES (A) AND (B) CHARACTERISTICS = CONCEPT AND ITS RANGE

   EXAMPLE
   "ONE TIME WHEN MY SUGAR WAS RUNNING 4+ I FELT REAL THIRSTY AND NERVOUS. ANOTHER TIME WHEN IT WAS 4+ I WAS THIRSTY, I URINATED A LOT AND HAD BLURRY VISION. I GUESS THAT ALL MUST GO WITH HAVING HIGH BLOOD SUGAR."

II SYMBOL FORMATION

1. EXPERIENCE, ACTION, OR EVENT + EXPERIENCE, ACTION, OR EVENT $\longrightarrow$ SYMBOL IS STATED ONLY
   (INTERNAL MANIFESTATIONS)　　　(EXTERNAL MANIFESTATIONS) $\quad$ PARTIALLY IN CONCRETE TERMS.

   EXAMPLE
   BODY MAKING TOO MUCH SUGAR + FEELING THIRSTY, $\longrightarrow$ DIABETES OR HIGH BLOOD
   URINATING A LOT, BEING HUNGRY $\qquad$ SUGAR

2. OBSERVED RELATIONSHIP + CONCRETE MANIFESTATION $\longrightarrow$ SYMBOL

   EXAMPLE
   FOOD INTAKE AND BLOOD SUGAR LEVEL + URINE TEST RESULTS $\longrightarrow$ 2+ MEANS WATCH MY DIET

III CLASSIFYING

DIFFERENCES IN EXTERNAL APPEARANCES OR IN INTERNAL STRUCTURE = DIFFERENCE IN THE STATE OF THE THING

EXAMPLES
"INSULIN WOULDN'T MIX WELL AND FELT THICKER WHEN I PULLED THE SYRINGE" = "INSULIN ISN'T NORMAL"
"TOE LOOKS ALL RIGHT BUT FEELS TENDER" = "TOE ISN'T NORMAL"

IV USING EXPERIENCE TO ARRIVE AT CONCEPT OR CATEGORIZE

REALITY
EXPERIENCE A AND/OR EXPERIENCE B AND/OR EXPERIENCE C = X

EXAMPLE
SHAKINESS WITH/OR WEAKNESS WITH/OR RACING HEART = HYPOGLYCEMIA

OPERATION AT THIS LEVEL
EXPERIENCE A	AT TIME 1	
EXPERIENCE B	AT TIME 2	A, B, C ARE RELATED
EXPERIENCE A AND C AT TIME 3	=	OR
EXPERIENCE A	AT TIME 4	A, B, C ARE X (HYPOGLYCEMIA)
EXPERIENCE C AND B AT TIME 5		

V RELATING EVENTS

REALITY
A + B + C $\qquad$ = X
(IN SOME QUANTITY + QUALITY)

EXAMPLES
1. "I STAY PRETTY NORMAL IF I EAT CLASS B VEGETABLES THREE TIMES A DAY AND MEAT TWICE A DAY "
2. "I STAY PRETTY NORMAL IF I EAT MEAT OR EGGS AT EACH MEAL BUT NO DESSERTS "
3. "WATER AND DIET SODAS AND COFFEE DON'T AFFECT MY BLOOD SUGAR LEVEL "

VI VIEWING SELF IN RELATION TO SITUATION

REALITY
1. EXPERIENCE OR STATE + PRESCRIBED RANGE OF X AND TECHNIQUE FOR REGULATING X = IDEAL OUTCOME
2. EXPERIENCE + JUDGMENT ABOUT AND WAY OF CARRYING OUT PRESCRIBED REGULATORY TECHNIQUE = ACTUAL OUTCOME

OPERATION AT THIS LEVEL
ABLE TO OPERATE IN LINE WITH REALITY, WITH THE EXCEPTION THAT THE KNOWLEDGE OF THE STATE WILL BE LIMITED BY THE LEVEL OF CONCEPTUALIZATION AND SYMBOLIZATION. IF THE TECHNIQUE INVOLVES A LARGE NUMBER OF FACTORS SOME MAY BE MISSED. THE LESS EXPLICIT ARE THE ONES LIKELY TO BE MISSED

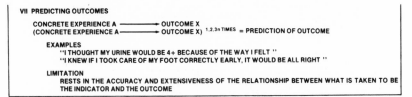

VII PREDICTING OUTCOMES

CONCRETE EXPERIENCE A ————→ OUTCOME X
(CONCRETE EXPERIENCE A————→ OUTCOME X) $^{1,2,3n\ TIMES}$ = PREDICTION OF OUTCOME

EXAMPLES
"I THOUGHT MY URINE WOULD BE 4+ BECAUSE OF THE WAY I FELT "
"I KNEW IF I TOOK CARE OF MY FOOT CORRECTLY EARLY, IT WOULD BE ALL RIGHT "

LIMITATION
RESTS IN THE ACCURACY AND EXTENSIVENESS OF THE RELATIONSHIP BETWEEN WHAT IS TAKEN TO BE
THE INDICATOR AND THE OUTCOME

Figure 8-6   Expressed inferences about seven types of intellectual operations characterized as focused on concrete or experienced wholes. (Courtesy of Joan E. Backscheider, R.N., Ph.D.)

In the previous chapter it was expressed that self-care agency is the power to engage in three sets of operations or processes (estimative, transitional, and productive), the power being comprised of ten abilities specific to the performance of the operations. According to this theoretic formulation, diagnosis of self-care agency would require the making of (1) observations of self-care operations engaged in or not engaged in by individuals or groups, and (2) observations to secure evidence upon which judgments can be based about the degree to which the ten abilities requisite to the performance of the operations are developed and operational.

Investigation of the human capabilities and dispositions foundational to self-care agency (Fig. 8-2) will provide nurses with the basis for making judgments about the point (within a range of points for each capability or disposition) at which the capability or disposition is operating. Particular operational values of these capabilities and dispositions will affect the operational level of self-care agency. Within an association frame of reference, the time-specific value of each capability or disposition affects the functional level of each of the ten abilities that are parts of the power element of self-care agency.

A schema showing three levels of organization as well as relationships among the elements of self-care agency, the foundational human capabilities and dispositions, and conditioning states and factors is presented in Figure 8-7. Nursing diagnosis can be started at any one of the three structural levels indicated in the figure. For example, on the basis of behavioral data, a nurse makes the judgment that an individual is comatose (arousal state, Level 3); the nurse then con-

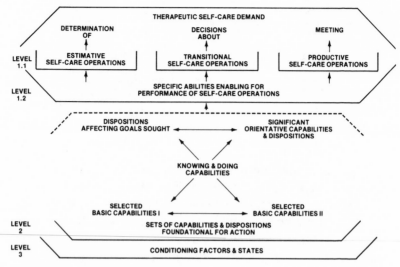

Figure 8-7 Three structural levels for diagnostic processes directed to the patient variable, self-care agency.

cludes that *self-care agency is not operational* because of interferences with attention and perception (Level 2, Selected Basic Capabilities II). Or a nurse makes the determination that a patient has made a number of errors in monitoring self for the effects and results of a self-care measure (Level 1.1). The diagnostic question now is why are the errors being made. Is it a failure on the part of the patient to maintain attention or exercise requisite vigilance (Level 1.2); or is it a limitation of one or more sensory exteroceptors (Level 2, Selected Basic Capabilities I); or a limitation of memory (Level 2, Selected Basic Capabilities II); or a limitation of motivation or orientation (Level 2)? A valid answer to the question *why are the errors being made* would express the power components of self-care agency or the capabilities or dispositions associated with the lack of effectiveness of the monitoring operations of the patient.

The schema presented in Figure 8-7 and the examples indicate that there is no single or simple approach to the diagnosis of self-care agency. Some inferences can be made on the basis of overt, readily available patient information;

or on the basis of data obtained by physicians for medical purposes. However, in making a definitive diagnosis of the self-care agency of an individual or group, the nurse must deal with the three named structural levels and the component parts of each level.

Research to further define and validate the theoretical and empirical formulations expressed in this and in the preceding chapter is needed.

REFERENCES

1. Backscheider, J. E.   The use of self as the essence of clinical supervision in ambulatory patient care. *Nurs. Clin. North Am.* 6:786–787, 1971.
2. Cousins, N.   Anatomy of an illness (as perceived by the patient). *N. Engl. J. Med.* 295:1458, 1976.
3. Lonergan, B. J. F.   *Insight.* New York: Philosophical Library, 1958. Pp. 280–283, 331.
4. Epstein, M. N., and Kaplan, E. B.   Criteria for Clinical Decision Making. In W. Schneider and A. L. Sågvall Hein (Eds.), *Computational Linguistics in Medicine.* Amsterdam and New York: North Holland Publishing, 1977. Pp. 35–44.
5. Nagel, E.   *The Structure of Science.* New York: Harcourt, Brace & World, 1961. Pp. 492–493.
6. Backscheider, J. E.   Self-care requirements, self-care capabilities, and nursing systems in the diabetic nurse management clinic. *Am. J. Public Health* 64:1138–1146, 1974.
7. Allport, G. W.   *Becoming.* New Haven: Yale University Press, 1955. Pp. 41–62.
8. Hebb, D. O.   Drives and the CNS (Conceptual Nervous System). In K. H. Pribram (Ed.), *Adaptation, Brain and Behavior 4.* Baltimore: Penguin, 1969. Pp. 180–183.
9. Mackworth, J. F.   *Vigilance and Habituation.* Baltimore: Penguin, 1969. Pp. 80–83.
10. Backscheider, J. E.   Unpublished data, 1971.
11. Orem, D. E.   *Nursing: Concepts of Practice.* New York: McGraw-Hill, 1971. P. 2.
12. Backscheider, J. E.   Personal account to D. E. Orem, 1971.
13. Backscheider, J. E.   Intellectual operations by stage of intellectual development (typewritten), 1970.
14. Backscheider, J. E.   Operational Level Knowing of a Diabetic Management Clinic Population (typewritten). Undated. Pp. 1, 4.

9

Nursing Knowledge and Nursing Practice

The provision of nursing to individuals and groups is a specialized type of practical endeavor. Like other human services, it involves practitioners in the acquisition and use of knowledge, in the creation of designs of the service to be produced to bring about specific effects and results, and in the deliberate performance of actions in such combinations and sequences that the service as designed or adjusted is provided and the results are achieved.

It is through the work of *practitioners of nursing* that the health service referred to in society as *nursing* is provided. Other roles (see Fig. 1-1) are enabling for or supportive of nursing practice. Different sets of goal orientations, action abilities, developed and perfected skills, and sustaining motives exist and operate in nurses prepared to engage effectively in nursing practice, scholarly advancement in nursing, research and development in nursing, theorizing toward the development and validation of explanatory systems in nursing, and teaching nursing. The theoretical construct *nursing agency* as used by NDCG members has as its referent the ability (i.e., power) of nurses to provide *nursing* to the public in jurisdictions where they can legitimately practice nursing. Each of the other named areas of endeavor in which nurses engage requires a different form of agency, which nurses form in themselves when they elect to function in one or a combination of the nonpractice roles.

As indicated in Figure 1-1, structured nursing knowledge descriptive and explanatory of the real world of nursing provides the organizing principle for the unification of the six named professional nurse roles. But it is the goal orientations of nurses functioning within the six roles (as well as their work operations) that serve as a fruitful base for their differentiation. The *practitioner* seeks to help the other, the patient, to achieve a result or results through *nursing.* The scholar seeks to move *self* to a *more advanced state of knowing* the practice discipline, *nursing.* The *theorist* seeks to *create explanations* that can be validated through research. The *developer* seeks to *discover and formalize ways and means to bring about specific types of nursing results* for persons who can benefit from nursing and to substantiate their *reliability* and *validity* through *research.* The *teacher* of nursing seeks to help the *other,* the nursing student, to develop the *power of nursing agency* and to begin to *form self as a nursing scholar.*

In summary, the practitioner and the teacher of nursing put nursing knowledge to use in serving the other. The scholar uses nursing knowledge already formalized and expressed to advance self to a higher level of knowing nursing. The theorist, the researcher, and the developer use existent knowledge to produce more knowledge, to validate knowledge, and to organize knowledge to express means (technologies) through which practical nursing results can be achieved. Theorists, researchers, and developers are producers of knowledge. Practitioners and teachers of nursing use nursing knowledge in serving others and, in doing so, may reach higher levels of understanding. But for all workers in nursing, it is the conditions of the members of a society, which can be regulated through nursing, that determine what needs to be done and what needs to be known through nursing.

This chapter is oriented to the knowing requirements of nurses engaged in nursing practice approaching the matter primarily from the perspective of the content of nurses' knowing operations. The chapter aims to set forth the kinds of knowledge that practitioners of nursing should have; illustrate ways of structuring existent knowledge to make it significant for purposes of nursing practice; give examples of the processes of model development helpful for nursing practice purposes; and finally to present some ideas about undergraduate nursing education, including an instructional system model in which nursing knowledge is described as an element of the system.

The chapter is viewed as helpful primarily in understanding the knowledge component of *nursing agency.* It should aid in understanding why the role of practitioner of nursing ideally should be combined with the role of nursing scholar.

THE KNOWING DIMENSION OF NURSING PRACTICE

In the practice of nursing, knowing, making, and doing operations are conjoined and integrated. In the mature nurse effective and firm habits facilitate these operations in ever new and changing situations of practice. However, the nursing student, the inexperienced nurse, and the teacher of nursing must come to understand the knowing, making, and doing operations of nursing as unique and separate but related operations. Since knowing is related to both making and doing (see Fig. 1-2) and takes place both prior in time and concurrently with them, attention is directed to this pivotal or central operation of nurses engaged in nursing practice.

Two Kinds of Knowledge

In situations of nursing practice, nurses relate to specific individuals or groups under their care. Nurses attend to persons under care with concern for the concrete and particular conditions and events that make these persons legitimate patients of nurses (p. 108). Nurses must determine *what these conditions and events are* and identify the factors that are in some way affecting their characteristics or occurrence. The knowledge gained by a nurse about the specific conditions, factors, and events and the relations among them is *empirical knowledge* of concrete situations of practice. The nurse moves self from a *condition of not knowing* a specific situation of practice to a *condition of having empirical knowledge* of it. To do this, nurses must be with, focus attention on, and make observations of persons under care and of existent environmental conditions.

A competent nurse's search for empirical knowledge in
specific situations of practice ends when the nurse is intellectually satisfied that the knowledge of the situation, which
has been attained at a point in time or over some duration of
time, is sufficient to answer questions of nursing practice; for
example, can this person be helped through nursing? or what
requirements for continuing care of self are being met, not
met at all, or inadequately met? or what role is the patient
capable of taking in self-care? If the nurse understands that
the level of knowing reached is inadequate for making nursing judgments and decisions in the situation, the search for
empirical knowledge should be continued. Thus *empirical
knowledge,* as the term is used here, is the content of nurses'
knowing concrete and particular conditions, factors, events,
or actions taken that are significant in nursing particular individuals or groups within particular environments.

This nursing practice requirement — that nurses have and
use empirical knowledge of situations of nursing practice in
designing and producing nursing — demands that nurses have
and use a second type of knowledge. This knowledge is referred to as *antecedent knowledge* because it must be existent
in the nurse prior to a nurse's seeking and having empirical
knowledge of specific situations of practice. Some types of
antecedent knowledge are enabling for a nurse to act to acquire empirical knowledge; other types are enabling for the
making and doing operations of nursing practice. Some antecedent knowledge is a product of life experiences of nurses.
But some is nursing-specific, requiring specialized education
for its mastery.

Empirical knowledge is concrete and specific to a situation
of practice; *antecedent knowledge is general.* Antecedent
knowledge may be factual, descriptive, or explanatory of
relations among existent entities; it may be statistical, based
on sequences of events and probabilities; or technological
(i.e., descriptive and explanatory of courses of actions as related to the bringing about of some range of effects and results under some range of conditions). Ideally, antecedent
knowledge of the nurse engaged in nursing practice is organized

into configurations that will facilitate its use. The formulation of such ideal configurations is an important responsibility of nurses in practice.

One concern of nurses in practice and in education has been the development of procedures for and the construction and validation of tools for use in collecting information about persons under care and the environmental conditions under which they live and function. But there is a related matter. This is the nature of the antecedent knowledge that nurses must have in order to go about acquiring empirical knowledge or to design and use tools to aid in information gathering. This matter is considered in the following section.

Qualitative Features of Antecedent Knowledge

To demonstrate the nature of knowledge that is referred to as *antecedent knowledge* (knowledge presupposed in the nurse prior to the nurse's engagement in the actions of nursing practice), one question that must be answered in all forms of practical endeavor is analyzed. The question selected for analysis is: *What is?* The results of the analysis provide the basis for making inferences about the kinds of antecedent knowledge that would exist in persons who are able to proceed to seek answers to this question in a range of types of practice situations.

The question *What is?* is examined within the frame of reference of human services. The results of the analysis can be generalized to all service situations. But the results are not at the level of generality that would be invariant for all occupations and professions. Within the frame of reference of human services, the analysis involves the following: (1) A setting forth of the human operations required to answer the broad question *What is?*; (2) listing the relevant subquestions that provide the basis for making inferences about the antecedent knowledge requirements of practitioners producing human services; and (3) inferring types of antecedent knowledge requirements.

The results of the analysis are presented in Table 9-1. All things being equal, the analysis substantiates the requirement

Table 9-1 Knowledge Requirements of Practitioners that are Antecedent to Answering the Question *What Is?*

Types of Human Operations	Requirements for Answering the Question *What Is?*		
	Subquestions to be Answered by the Practitioner	Antecedent Knowledge Requirements of Practitioners
Directing, focusing, and maintaining attention	What conditions and factors existent in the other reveal a need that can be met by this human service?	Descriptions and explanations of the human condition(s) that legitimate a relation between the producer of a human service and persons served
	To what should attention be directed?	The human and environmental phenomena from which such conditions can be inferred
	How can and should the producer of the service be physically located and positioned in relation to the person or group served?	The nature and the range of forms in which the service can be produced
Making observations	What can be observed in the situation where service is to be produced? What should be observed? When? For what time duration?	The sensible characteristics of sets of phenomena
		The nature and frequency of change to be expected
	What perceptual strategies are useful in (1) making observations of static conditions, events, or deliberate actions performed; and (2) discovery of high-order structures?	The meaning of change
		Reliable and valid perceptual strategies that can give form to observational technologies and perceptual skills
		The nature and form of the data

Identifying and understanding the data	What modes of data collection should be used? What unities can be grasped in the structure and details of the data? What relations can be grasped among the different kinds of data? What concepts will subsume the data?	Data collection methodologies and tools that have utility in recording and organizing data Valid and organized descriptive and explanatory knowledge of the entities under observation
Characterizing that which has been identified	What characterizing judgments can be made about the observed entities on the basis of the quality and quantity of data obtained?	The quality of the data required for making judgments about conditions and happenings
Expressing characterizing judgments	How can a judgment(s) be formulated and expressed to accurately characterize conditions, factors, events, or courses of action about which data was obtained?	Rules for the selection and organization of words in expressing characterizing judgments Terms that are descriptive of observable entities and high-order structures
Appraising that which has been observed and characterized	What meaning is conveyed by the existence of the characterized entities?	The fit of the characterized entity into the schema of human structure and functioning or the schema of the human environment

Table 9-1 (continued)

Types of Human Operations	Subquestions to be Answered by the Practitioner	Antecedent Knowledge Requirements of Practitioners
Expressing appraising judgments	How can this meaning be formulated and expressed as an appraising judgment?	Rules for the selection and organization of words in expressing appraising judgments
		Terms that express the human meaning of conditions, and so forth, about which observations can be made

for antecedent knowledge in producers of human services and sets forth the nature and form of the knowledge that is antecedent to a practitioner's engagement in answering the question: What is existent in this practice situation? The same type of analysis can be done with respect to the further practice questions *What can be?* and *What should be?* and for the making and doing operations through which human services are produced.

The mastery of knowledge that is presupposed in nurses prior to actual engagement in nursing practice is one result sought by nursing students and by nurses in practice through engagement in scholarly pursuit of nursing as a discipline of knowledge. This book was designed and developed to express the understandings of one group of nurses about the nature and form of antecedent knowledge essential for nurses engaged in nursing practice and to support and encourage the engagement of nurses in the further structuring of nursing knowledge. Reflection will reveal that some of the antecedent knowledge requirements identified in Table 9-1 have been formulated and expressed in Chapters 5 through 8. This knowledge is general, abstract, and invariant for situations of practice.

One essential component of a nurse's antecedent knowledge is a general concept of nursing that specifies the proper object of nursing as well as its form and content. Nurses who deliberately select a general concept of nursing with an interest in increasing their understanding of nursing sometimes initiate a process of reexamination of the structure of nursing knowledge and of nursing practice (their own and that of others) in reality situations. This process moves a nurse into a position of examining and attempting to position within the selected concept of nursing the complexities of the world in which nurses practice nursing. The nurse who moves to this point in the process of reexamination assumes the position of validator and developer of the general concept selected. Two questions now become of major concern to the nurse:

1. Does the general concept of nursing provide dimensions for a way of structuring nursing in reality situations that specifies and enhances opportunities to provide effective nursing services to patients?

2. How can the general concept of nursing or the substantive structure of its elements be refined to take into account more of the complexities of nursing in reality situations?

Since the inception of the Group as the Nursing Model Committee, some members of the NDCG have dealt with reality nursing situations as sources of boundary material to establish the dimensions of an adequate and valid general concept of nursing. Since the inception of the NDCG, some of the members have maintained themselves in positions in which they could have control over the design and development of nursing systems in health-care institutions with inpatient and outpatient services. In these positions NDCG members have been able to address problems related to the adequacy of the general concept of nursing in use by the Group for (1) structuring nursing systems, (2) identifying specific factors or conditions that further define nursing variables, their ranges of variances, and their subjectivity to control measures, and (3) exploring methods appropriate for the study of nursing practice.

A PRACTITIONER'S USE OF NURSING CONCEPTS

The work of NDCG members in nursing practice situations has been and is producing evidence to support the *utility* as well as reliability and validity of the concepts of nursing and nursing system. The subsequent description of one practice situation illustrates a nurse's use of the NDCG concept of *nursing system.*

Designing a Nursing System

An experience of one NDCG member[1] in a first encounter with a patient (a woman, 60 years of age, hospitalized because of injuries resulting from a fall in her home) provided clear-cut data that could be structured from the perspective of the Group's concept of nursing. The data sought and ac-

[1] Sheila M. McCarthy

cumulated by the nurse and her nursing judgments were the bases for her design for a system of roles, relationships, and activities to guide the endeavors of the nurse and the patient.

Operating within the framework of the Group's concept of nursing with its specific conceptual elements, the nurse accepted the following:

1. The system set up between her and the patient would be an *action system* oriented to and designed around the patient's requirements for therapeutic self-care and the patient's self-care agency.
2. The patient would be experiencing demands for self-care resulting from her injury and its treatment and also from the elements of the system of health-related self-care she routinely performed.
3. The nurse must define nurse- and patient-contributed actions toward meeting the patient's requirements for therapeutic self-care; the nurse's contributions would be dependent on the patient's capacities to engage in required activities.
4. A valid system of nursing assistance related to the existence in the patient of a self-care deficit cannot be initiated until the reasons for, and type and amount of, nursing assistance needed by the patient are identified and described through an assessment process.
5. As nurse, one's capabilities are requisite for (and exceed the demands of) this situation.

In accepting the above assumptions, the nurse is taking a position on conditions in patients that validate her work in society and on the nature of the broadest generalizations that will serve her in the collection, interpretation, and organization of data within the boundaries of a nursing focus. The question with which she deals is this: What specific reality in the form of events will emerge when I utilize my concept of nursing in the care of this specific patient?

Given the conceptual structure and the reality elements expressed in the five assumptions, the nurse made use of resources available to her (the medical record, nursing personnel, physicians) and then entered into her initial contact with the patient for purposes of answering the questions: Why does Mrs. X need nursing and what would be appropriate nursing services for her today and for some longer period of time?

Assessment　Information highlighting a nursing focus for this 60-year-old hospitalized woman is presented in outline form under four headings.

I. The Health Deviation and Its Medical Management
   A. *Condition.* Injuries from a fall down steps; cause of fall unknown. Multiple bruises; lumbar injury — fracture first vertebra; questionable intracranial lesion — neurologic findings negative; head wound — sutured laceration of scalp (small)
   B. *Medical therapy*
      1. Medication for
         a. Pain
         b. Relief of skeletal muscle spasm and reduction of tension
      2. Restriction of activity
         a. Bed rest
         b. Limitation in movement in bed
         c. Brace for back
      3. Heat treatments to back (hydroculator packs)
   C. *Outcome.* Probable return to normal or near normal functioning after period of restricted activity
II. General Health Status: Good, with consideration to be given to aging process
III. Patient's Perspectives and Concerns — present condition, general health state, self-care, expressed concerns
   A. *Therapeutic regimen*
      1. Movement. Muscle aches and stiffness. Difficulty in movement when raising shoulder from the bed. Patient knew that her doctor would allow her to sit up. The nurse reviewed the movements she could perform. The patient knew why she would have to wear a brace (for fractured vertebra).
      2. Medications. Patient stated she believed in medications. "I am a homeopath at heart." She said she liked the pain medication because it took away the pain without making her groggy. She said she was taking no medications at home.
   B. *Some usual self-care practices*
      1. Diet. Thinks diet is very important. Never eats spicy foods; recognizes the value of vitamins and proteins; orange juice contains vitamin C; drinking water facilitates bowel movements; milk contains calcium.
      2. Activity. Her husband and she like to keep active and healthy.
      3. Bathing. Patient was concerned about inability to bend to shave her legs; usually did this every two days; keeps legs tanned and lubricated with creams. Patient analyzed with

the nurse what parts of the bath she could perform for herself — face, arms, and anterior trunk; patient preferred to do her own bathing as much as possible.
C. *Aging*
Concern with aging. Patient commented, "We should all be concerned about geriatrics."
D. *Personal and social*
1. Activities. Described activities: those enjoyed with her husband; going to hairdresser; restaurants enjoyed for good foods; and reasonable costs for both. Distressed over missed hairdresser appointment. Likes to look attractive to please her husband
2. Future plans. Plan to retire in a southern state where she and her husband own a house
3. Family. Told about her house and children, now married. Told about one in another country whom she had visited. Expressed concern about sanitary conditions there
IV. Patient Interviews the Nurse
Questions: Asked how long the nurse had lived in the local area, preferred places to eat, and so on
V. Nurse's Judgments Relevant to Patient as Self-Care Agent — based on the information cited as well as other information
A. The patient has a strong self-care system directed to keeping "young" and "strong."
B. The patient's usual self-care system is tied in with that of her husband.
C. The patient's self-care system is tied into her system of beliefs about health and about naturopathy and homeopathy.
D. The patient lives a patterned life.
E. The patient has understanding of, as well as questions about the demands for, self-care and effects on one's self-care system when living outside the United States.
F. The patient has awareness of medical orders and of ways to restrict movement. Has knowledge of the pathology of her case.
G. Limitations exist in relation to movements or actions requiring body flexibility. These limitations result in a deficit in being able to execute some self-care measures and activities of her system of living.
H. The patient has a need to discuss potential implications of outcomes of her present state for her system of living.

Nursing Assistance   As a result of nursing judgments about the dimensions of the patient's self-care agency, the following judgments about patient and nurse roles in the patient's continuing care were made:

1. The patient is director of her own universal self-care with the assistance of the professional nurse. This means that the nurse must permit the patient to follow her usual self-care practices except as they require adjustment to her limitations of movement and to prevent possible further damage through movement.
2. The nurse performs certain measures for the patient in relation to (a) maintaining cleanliness of the area of the scalp lacerations, and (b) monitoring vital signs and neurologic signs.
3. The nurse provides for the assistance necessary to accomplish (a) bathing and grooming, (b) turning, (c) communication of symptoms experienced by the patient to other nurses and physicians, (d) periodic heat treatments with precautions to prevent burns, and (e) the prescribed pharmacotherapy.
4. The nurse provides the supportive assistance needed for the patient to (a) adjust her self-image, (b) restrict her movements, and (c) adjust to hospitalization.
5. The nurse provides educative assistance related to potential immediate and long-range implications of various outcomes of her injuries as these are related to self-care and system of living. Particular instruction is given with regard to the patient's safe use of hydroculator packs after discharge.

The judgments about nurse role and patient role in the nursing situation led to the conclusion that the action system that would emerge from nurse- and patient-role performance would have the structure of a partly compensatory system of nursing assistance [1]. In the reality situation, patient and nurse did perform within the roles delineated by the NDCG member.

Effects on the General Concept of Nursing
This instance of nursing practice was discussed and analyzed in an NDCG conference and is viewed as instrumental in the isolation and development of the substantive structure of the element, *self-care agency*. Members were able to form conceptualizations of component parts of the element, self-care agency, and relations among the parts. Other insights included (1) a relation between self-image and a person's view

of self as self-care agent; (2) relations between the medical regimen instituted and patient's concerns, either about meeting specific care requirements or about their effects on the system of self-care and daily living; and (3) patient's expressed concerns and actions as evidence of limitations to engage in self-care.

Products of this work session were two models: one was specific to the patient under discussion (Fig. 9-1); the other was an *initial nursing approach* model useful in any nursing situation (see Chap. 6, pp. 172—173). These models are guides for NDCG members to explore the dimensions of nursing situations and to develop and use nursing assessment guides.

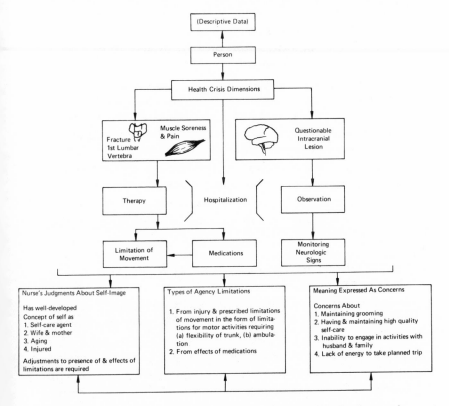

Figure 9-1   Descriptive data and nursing judgments organized around focuses.

Further discussion of this instance of nursing practice led to the development of the model shown in Figure 6-12. Discussions also involved exploration of the range over which a *partly compensatory nursing system* could vary — moving closer at one extreme of its range to the *wholly compensatory nursing system* and at the other extreme to the *supportive-educative* type nursing system.

Reflection on this situation reveals that *nursing agency* was deliberately related to the patient (1) as injured, (2) as suffering from and living with effects of the injury, and (3) as having a life style and a self-care system both of which are relevant to the patient's interest in, willingness to, and readiness to enter into and contribute to a temporarily changed life style and self-care system. The nursing agency of the nurse is the critical element determining whether the nurse can involve the patient; afford the patient her proper role in the situation (as delineated by objective data); and provide the input required for the production of nursing assistance over time.

Situations such as that just discussed need to be analyzed from the perspective of levels of expectations and responsibilities for types of practitioners. Ultimately this would lead to the design of a system of care for the patient describing the contributions of various levels of workers. The responsibilities attached to the nurse at each level would then provide structuring data for education in various types of programs.

THE STRUCTURE OF ANTECEDENT NURSING KNOWLEDGE

Because of the diversity and complexity of nursing cases, NDCG members have been attentive to the need to structure existent knowledge in forms useful to nurses engaged in nursing practice. Nursing cases can be grouped on the basis of resemblances among them. As a genus within instances of occurrence of requirements for human services, nursing cases should be understood and can be classified in terms of differences in ends sought and differences in the actions required to achieve the ends. Knowledge that is antecedent to nurses' engagement in nursing practice should be structured to make these differences explicit.

One position to be taken is that antecedent knowledge should be organized and expressed according to degrees of invariance with respect to instances of individual and group health-care requirements that can be met through nursing. As previously stated, some antecedent knowledge is invariant for all nursing cases but other antecedent knowledge is invariant for some range of types of nursing cases when specific factors are exercising a conditioning influence on the nursing system variables.

Three examples of NDCG members' endeavors to structure antecedent knowledge required by nurses are presented. All the examples assume the acceptance and use by NDCG members of (1) self-care deficit as explanatory of why individuals require nursing; (2) nursing systems as products designed and produced by nurses to achieve nursing goals; and (3) the conceptual constructs, therapeutic self-care demand, self-care agency, and nursing agency, viewed as qualities of persons, qualities that operate as variables within the technologic subsystems of nursing systems. The examples differ in focus and in scope. All are illustrative of the effort and the nature of the work involved in the structuring of knowledge that is antecedent to nursing practice.

Nursing System Variables and Cerebrovascular Accidents
An effort was made by Hartnett-Rauckhorst in 1977 to 1978 to organize (i.e., structure) knowledge about cerebrovascular accidents derived from the fields of neurophysiology, pathology, medicine, psychology, sociology, nursing, and physical and occupational therapy around the nursing system variables, therapeutic self-care demand, self-care agency, and nursing agency. The occurrence of a stroke was viewed as a basic conditioning factor that sets up the requirement for development of a nursing system. This is an example of bringing together existing knowledge derived from the literature of nursing and nursing-related fields into a nursing frame-

work and of applying the NDCG's theory of nursing system to a particular patient population.

From the perspectives of pathology and medicine, a cerebrovascular accident or a stroke is the cardinal feature of cerebrovascular diseases. A stroke is the sudden development of a *focal neurologic deficit* resultant from the *effects* of *pathologic processes in one or more blood vessels* of the brain *on brain tissue.* Cerebrovascular accidents range in degree from very severe to very mild. The occurrence of a cerebrovascular accident and the time sequential occurrence of subsequent events are referred to as the *time profile* or the *stages of cerebrovascular accidents.*

Five stages were utilized in the work of organizing existent knowledge about stroke around the nursing system variables. These stages are referred to as:

Stage I   Being at risk for cerebrovascular accidents or having premonitory signs

Stage II   Acute stage of a cerebrovascular accident (severe stroke)
             A. Unconscious phase
             B. Returning consciousness phase

Stage III   Convalescent stage of cerebrovascular accidents

Stage IV   Rehabilitation stage following cerebrovascular accidents

Stage V   Health maintenance or continuing care stage following cerebrovascular accidents

In using the foregoing time dimensions that mark the patterns of occurrence of types of events and results associated with stroke, it is important to understand that for particular individuals the time profile need not extend over the five stages. For example, some persons at risk (Stage I) do not have cerebrovascular accidents; individuals may die in the acute stage (Stage II), or the stroke may be mild rather than severe; or individuals may be arrested in Stage III, not able to progress to Stage IV or to Stage V.

The results of knowledge structuring using the selected basic conditioning factor, cerebrovascular accident, were formulated and are presented as (1) a charting of the degrees of operability of self-care agency by stages of cerebrovascular accidents; (2) an example of the demand for the operation of self-care agency associated with one stage of stroke, Stage I; (3) descriptive models of the characteristics of the nursing system variables by stages of cerebrovascular accidents; and (4) a charting of variations in nursing goals, nursing systems, and nursing roles in the five stages of cerebrovascular accidents.

These models are an initial attempt to organize knowledge about cerebrovascular accidents around the NDCG's conceptualizations of nursing system variables. They provide a basis for further study and refinement of the characteristics and components of the nursing system variables at each stage of stroke. Valid and reliable assessment tools for gathering evidence about nursing system variables can then be developed. This evidence would contribute to the development of a body of theoretical knowledge descriptive and explanatory of the nursing system variables at each stage of stroke. It would also provide a basis for the development of a body of practical knowledge that can provide guidance and direction to nurses who are confronted with questions of practice regarding the design and the delivery of nursing care to persons at each stage of stroke.

Operability of Self-Care Agency   Following strokes, there can be a great variation of effects on the power components of self-care agency, since the effects of strokes on human functioning vary over a wide range.

The medical literature reports effects of stroke in terms of signs and symptoms and the anatomic structures involved. On the basis of signs and symptoms identified in the literature, judgments were made about their association with "human capabilities and dispositions" requisite for engagement in self-care (see Fig. 8-2). On the basis of these judgments inferences were made about how the degree of operability of self-care agency could be affected in each stage of stroke. The following diagram represents the progression of knowing and the conceptual constructs used.

| Having knowledge of signs and symptoms of cerebrovascular accidents | → | Having insights and making judgments about associations of signs and symptoms with human capabilities and dispositions basic to human action | → | Making inferences about degree of operability of the power components of self-care agency by stages of cerebrovascular accidents |

The progression of knowing illustrated in the diagram and the use of the literature as the resource for obtaining knowledge of signs and symptoms of stroke parallel the progression of knowing of nurses in practice who must identify and then attach nursing meaning to the concrete and particular signs and symptoms of individual patients.

The common and gross patterns of operability of self-care agency associated with the stages of cerebrovascular accident are shown in Table 9-2. The degrees of operability of self-care agency are indicated by the terms *fully operative, partially operative,* and *not operative.* Table 9-2 should be read with the understanding that the represented patterns of operability of self-care agency are inferences about the effects and results of cerebrovascular accidents on the operability of each power component of self-care agency. In concrete situations of nursing practice, other factors may be conditioning one or more of the power components.

Table 9-2 does not express patterns of adequacy of self-care agency as related to a therapeutic self-care demand. For example, power components of self-care agency may be fully operative in Stage I but not adequately developed in relation to specific self-care operations. This is demonstrated in the following section.

New Demands for Self-Care Operations, Stage I   Being at risk for a cerebrovascular accident operates as a factor that changes the objective value of an individual's *therapeutic self-care demand.* New self-care requirements arise or there is need for adjustments in existent requirements. The self-care requirements occasioned by being at risk for stroke increase

Table 9-2   Common Patterns of Operability of Self-Care Agency Associated with the Five Stages of Cerebrovascular Accidents

Power Components of Self-Care Agency	Patterns of Operability Cerebrovascular Accident Stages				
	I [a]	II	III	IV [a]	V [a]
1. Maintenance of attention and vigilance	FO	NO/PO	PO	PO	PO/FO
2. Controlled use of available physical energy	FO	NO	NO/PO	PO	PO/FO
3. Control of position of body and its parts in execution of movements	FO	NO/PO	NO/PO	PO	PO/FO
4. Reasoning within a self-care frame of reference	FO	NO/PO	NO/PO	NO/PO	PO/FO
5. Motivations or goal orientations to self-care	FO	NO	NO/PO	PO/FO	PO/FO
6. Decision-making about care of self	FO	NO	NO/PO	PO/FO	PO/FO
7. Acquiring, retaining, operationalizing technical knowledge about self-care	FO	NO	NO/PO	PO	PO/FO
8. Having repertoire of self-care skills	FO	NO	NO/PO	PO	PO/FO
9. Ordering discrete self-care actions	FO	NO	NO/PO	PO	PO/FO
10. Integrating self-care operations with other aspects of daily living	FO	NO	NO/PO	PO	PO/FO

[a] Fully operative means operation is *unaffected* by the cerebrovascular accident.
Key: FO = Fully operative; PO = partially operative; NO = not operative; / = or.

the demand on an individual both for the exercise of self-care agency and for its further development. This is a different situation from those that exist during and following the occurrence of a stroke. In these later situations the *demand* for the *exercise for self-care agency is increased* at the same time that the *power components of self-care agency* are rendered *not operative* or *partly operative* by the effects of the stroke.

The following is an example of new courses of self-care actions that are required if the condition of "being at risk for cerebrovascular accidents" is to be regulated. New estimative, transitional, and productive self-care operations contribute to meeting the self-care requirements for "prevention of hazards" and "being normal" [1, pp. 26–28].

New Estimative Self-Care Operations and Results

1. Investigation of the aging process and associated risk factors, especially factors that increase risk of stroke (e.g., age, weight, life-style, and habits; stress hypertension, diabetes, arteriosclerosis)
   Result. Acquired technical knowledge that points to the need for periodic health checkups and use of valid means of control of risk factors
2. Investigation (including health evaluation) to become aware of those internal and external factors that increase risk for stroke that are probably operational in self
   Result. Knowledge of factors that are or could be putting self at risk for stroke

Associated Transitional Operations and Results

1a. Reflecting on the technical knowledge acquired to determine the course of action to be followed
   Result. Judgments about the need for periodic health checkups, the best place to secure them, and the best time for them
1b. Deciding about what will be done with respect to periodic health checkups
   Result. Decision to have or not to have periodic health checkups
2a. Reflecting on empirical knowledge of self and those internal and external factors that are probably making one at risk for stroke
   Result. Judgment that self is at *high* or *low risk* for stroke

2b. Deciding what courses of action to follow with respect to regulation of risk factors
      Result. Decisions about following or not following courses of action that will or will not keep risk factors under a degree of control

Associated Productive Operations and Results

1a. Make and keep appointments for periodic health checkups
1b. Actively participate in the procedures associated with each health checkup
1c. Receive information from each health checkup
      Result. Having information about health state
2a. Engage in regulatory actions to reduce risk of stroke
2b. Monitor self for own performance of regulatory actions and for evidence of effects and results of the action
      Result. Knowledge that self-care requirements are being met with some degree of effectiveness or are not being met; knowledge of the presence or absence of evidence of the effects and results of the courses of action taken to meet self-care requirements

An application of the foregoing is expressed in relation to a 34-year-old woman.

As a result of the *estimative* self-care operations, a 34-year-old woman with a family history of hypertension and stroke who is 15 pounds overweight will gain empirical and experiential knowledge of known risk factors and how they constitute a threat to her life and health and a realization that some of these factors (e.g., weight and blood pressure) can be modified to reduce the risk. She recognizes that diet modification (in terms of calories and sodium intake) is an effective means available to regulate existing risk factor(s). As a result of *transitional* self-care operations, this woman judges that she should modify her diet and decides that she will perform the regulatory self-care operations this entails. As a result of *productive* self-care operations, this woman will have learned what foods are high and low in calories and sodium, developed a diet plan and menus, and planned for food buying and preparation. Within a daily and weekly time frame she will buy, prepare, and eat a diet lower in calories and sodium. She will monitor food labels, size of portions, cooking procedures (especially if prepared by others), and check her weight regularly to obtain data about whether she is losing weight at a safe rate or whether weight loss is not being achieved. She will ascertain her blood pressure reading at each contact with health professionals. She will reflect on the evidence of the results and decide whether to continue with the present diet modification, to adapt it further, or to discontinue it.

This example of how "being at risk for stroke" generates new self-care requirements to be met through new self-care operations is further elaborated in the following analysis.

Changing Values of Nursing System Variables   Six models were developed to express in a modified way the range over which the values of the two patient variables (therapeutic self-care demand and self-care agency) are known to vary and the range over which the nurse variable (nursing agency) should vary during the stages of stroke. Components of the *therapeutic self-care demand* associated with stroke are expressed as *courses of action* that should ideally be performed. Limitations of *self-care agency* are expressed in terms of inappropriate courses of self-care action commonly taken or as inadequate power components of self-care agency or as interferences with the basic capabilities or dispositions for self-care. Components of *nursing agency* are expressed as kinds of knowledge and skills. The knowledge expressed in the models in relation to three nursing system variables was extracted from the literature and *should not be considered as necessarily complete, definitive, or precisely organized.*

The models include expressions about the populations to be served and general goals for health care for these populations (goals common to all persons involved). Levels of prevention of disease and injury were used to express general goals for health care. The levels of prevention paradigm proved useful in organizing the material within the sequential stages of cerebrovascular accident, a pathophysiologic event.

Prior to the onset of a stroke, the focus is on primary prevention for the entire community and secondary prevention for individuals with high-risk profiles or with evidence of premonitory signs. During the acute, convalescent, and rehabilitative stages, the main focus is on tertiary prevention with concern for primary and secondary prevention in terms of preventing the onset or minimizing the effects of new pathologic changes. In the health maintenance or the continuing care stage, the main focus is on secondary prevention with continued concern for both primary prevention of new pathologic changes and tertiary prevention in terms of continuing restorative and rehabilitative goals.

During the development of the models, it became clear that the demand on nurses to think using particular combinations of views of man varies with the stages of stroke. In Stages I and V there is a demand on the nurse to think primarily within the combination of person-agent-symbolizer-organism views and, in a more limited way, to think within the view of *object* (i.e., man) subject to physical forces. In Stage II, thought processes move within the organism-object combination and within the person-agent-symbolizer combination in relation to achieving goals of primary and secondary prevention.

Development of these models involved thinking in the person, agency, and action frames of reference (see Fig. 7-2). In the *person* frame of reference a range of life-styles and habits were seen as indicative of states not enabling for deliberate action in the prestroke phase. The acute phase of stroke (in severe strokes) was seen as putting the person in a state that is completely nonenabling for deliberate action. In the convalescent and rehabilitation phases, the person was seen as being in a series of states which were partially and progressively more enabling for action. In the *agency* frame of reference, self-care agency is considered from the viewpoint of self-care agency limitations, which are expressed at (1) the level of self-care actions, (2) the more basic level of power components of self-care agency, or (3) the foundational level of human capabilities and dispositions basic to engagement in self-care.

It is grossly evident from the models that the operability and redevelopment of self-care agency can vary greatly in the various stages of cerebrovascular accident. The type or degree of self-care deficit that can exist at each stage of stroke and because of the stroke is indicated. A self-care deficit as a nursing diagnosis means that self-care agency is inadequate to meet the therapeutic self-care demand. In the *action* frame of reference, the therapeutic self-care demand expresses the self-care actions required to maintain and promote life and health at each stage. These discrete self-care actions would have to be organized within the more comprehensive self-care system.

As indicated, the organization of knowledge extracted from the literature around the nursing system variables is the result of an initial effort. If the paradigms are useful they can serve as guides for the further structuring and refinement of this area of knowledge.

DESCRIPTIVE MODELS OF NURSING SYSTEM VARIABLES IN THE STAGES OF CEREBROVASCULAR ACCIDENT

Stage I Being at Risk for Cerebrovascular Accidents or Having Premonitory Signs

Population. Individuals with high risk for cerebrovascular accidents or with premonitory signs. The community as a whole

Health Care Goals
Secondary Prevention
↕
Primary Prevention

Components of the Therapeutic Self-Care Demand
Seeking of regular health checkups

Types of Self-Care Agency Limitations
Seeking of only episodic health care

Acknowledgment of risk profile

Ignorance of risk factors and effective preventive measures

Adaptations of life-style to reduce risk

Denial of threat presented by the risk profile

Lack of motivation to change lifestyle

When the above named self-care agency limitations are existent, there will be a partial self-care deficit.

Components of Nursing Agency
Theoretical Knowledge of
  Stroke risk factors and premonitory signs
    Normal parameters of variables reflecting risk of stroke (e.g., blood pressure, weight)
    Patterns of health behavior of individuals, small groups, communities

Teaching-learning theory
Theory and strategies of change
Skills for
Health assessment screening, case-finding, referral, and follow-up of
high risk individuals
Assessment of population groups re: risk profile characteristics and
community resources
Public relations
Community planning
Preparation and use of media of mass communication
Teaching and support of individuals and groups
Stage II Acute Stage of Cerebrovascular Accident
A. Unconscious Phase (Severe Stroke)

Population. Individuals who have had a severe stroke recently

Health Care Goals

Tertiary Prevention

Primary
Prevention ⟷ Secondary
Prevention

Components of the Therapeutic Self-Care Demand

Modification of entire range of universal self-care requirements

Frequent monitoring of multiple physiologic variables

Administration and monitoring of effects of specific drugs (e.g., antihypertensives, anticoagulants)

Detection and management of life-threatening complications (e.g., shock, hyperthermal convulsions)

Types of Self-Care Agency Limitations

Lack of awareness of environment and inoperative mental processes

Inoperative protective reflexes

Immobility (with its range of hazards to the structural and functional integrity of the organism)

Self-care agency will be *not operative* in persons who have had severe strokes, and the deficit for engagement in self care will be complete qualitatively and quantitatively.

Components of Nursing Agency
Theoretical knowledge of
Pathophysiology of stroke
Normal parameters and interrelationships of variables reflecting
health state; deviations from the norm that require immediate
referral and action
Effects and consequences of immobility

Causes and effects of unconscious state

Rationale for and therapeutic and untoward effects of medical. treatment modalities

Crisis and crisis intervention theory

Skills for or in the nature of

Techniques for meeting universal self-care requirements (to maintain circulation and oxygenation of tissues, nutrition and fluid balance, musculoskeletal integrity, skin and mucous membrane integrity, elimination, a balance of rest and sensory social stimulation, and safety of environment) in unconscious individual

Assessment of family's level of coping

Crisis intervention techniques

Assessment of neurologic status and other body systems reflecting health state

Administration of special treatment modalities (e.g., hypothermia)

Recognition of condition changes that indicate life-threatening emergencies and require immediate intervention or referral

Designing, operationalizing, and managing complex wholly compensatory nursing systems through which the universal and health deviation self-care requirements within the therapeutic self-care demand are integrated and met through nurse action

B. Phase of Returning Consciousness (Severe Stroke)

Population. Individuals who recently sustained a stroke and who are not yet medically stable but are regaining consciousness	*Health Care Goals* As in Phase A
Components of the Therapeutic Self-Care Demand	*Types of Self-Care Agency Limitations*
Self-monitoring and universal self-care modifications still required as in Stage II A with reemergence of need to be normal	Mental confusion, memory gaps, and/or emotional lability (that will impair judgment and decision-making)
Reorientation of self to persons, places, things in environment	Denial of paralysis; neglect of affected side
Acknowledgment of changes in self	Some combination of sensory, perceptual, motor, and communication (language) impairments)
Reestablishment of communication systems	

Beginning resumption of aspects of integrated human
functioning requisite to
self-care agency (e.g., decision-making)
Cooperation with performance
of measures of care asso-
ciated with the therapeu-
tic modalities
Avoiding activities that may
increase intracranial pressure
Extensive deficit for engagement in self-care due to the stroke. Extent of self-care deficit varies with severity of the stroke.
Components of Nursing Agency
Theoretical Knowledge
    All types required for Stage II A plus
    Usual patterns of recovery from stroke and of return to conscious
       state
    Theory concerning human sensation, perception, cognition, mem-
       ory, emotion, motivation; body- and self-image, experience of
       loss, and stages of the grieving process
    Major types of sensory, perceptual, cognitive, emotional, motor,
       and communication deficits that occur following stroke
Skills
    All types required for Stage II A plus
    Assessment of signs of returning consciousness and types and
       severity of deficits for action
    Reorientation and remotivation techniques
    Assessment of signs of readiness to participate in self-care and/or
       contraindications to increasing participation
    Establishment of communication systems and supportive inter-
       personal environments
Stage III Convalescent Stage of Cerebrovascular Accident

Population. Individuals who have survived acute stage and whose medically defined condition has stabilized

Health Care Goals
(Rehabilitation)
Tertiary Prevention

Primary Prevention ←→ Secondary Prevention

Components of the Therapeutic Self-Care Demand
Need to be normal requires in-
creasing participation in ac-

Types of Self-Care Agency Limitations
Residual neurological deficits become more clearly defined re:

tivities of daily living to meet universal self-care requirements

Expending effort to pay attention to and to perform initial rehabilitative tasks

Coping with changes in self (body and self-image, dependency, role loss) with hope for functional improvement and acknowledgment of own role in this

Reestablishment of relationships with family or loved ones

Working for limited, short-term goals with tolerance for slow progress or setbacks

Coping with persistence of bowel and/or bladder incontinence

Learning to relate to affected side and use it in accomplishing self-care (if possible)

Development of realistic goals that have meaning for self

how they affect self-care agency. For example: hemianopsia (unaware of things in one-half of visual field); distortion of depth perception and of vertical-horizontal planes (balance problems, bumps into things, drops things); short attention span, persisting disorientation or memory gaps; continued denial of or development of depressive reaction to changes in self; paralysis, weakness, and/or spasticity of muscles on affected side; aphasia (receptive and/or expressive) or dysarthria

Extensive deficit for engagement in self-care due to the stroke. Extent of the deficit varies with the severity of the stroke.

Components of Nursing Agency

Theoretical Knowledge

All types required for Stage II B plus

Phases of recovery and potential ranges of functional return from common neurologic deficits after stroke

Functions and goals of the rehabilitative therapies (occupational, physical, and speech)

Ways to compensate for or minimize effects of various neurologic deficits

Teaching-learning of neurologically impaired

Normal adult growth and development

Skills

All types required for Stage II B plus

Ability to shift from predominantly "doer" to "observer-teacher" role

Coordination of supportive-developmental or partly compensatory
nursing system with rehabilitative therapies

Assessment of developmental status and response to losses of function and roles

Techniques to compensate for neurologic deficits and promote return of function

Techniques for teaching neurologically impaired

Stage IV Rehabilitation Stage of Cerebrovascular Accident

Population. Individuals whose action deficits are established and potential for restoration of function largely predictable	*Health Goals* As in Stage III
Components of the Therapeutic Self-Care Demand	*Types of Self-Care Limitations*
Same as for Stage III but with increased focus on need to be normal and to resume usual activities of daily living and life roles (to extent possible)	Same as for Stage III
Learning how to monitor own health state and to incorporate rehabilitative and medical regimen requirements into self-care system	Number and severity of the limitations vary with each individual and with right- and left-sided cerebrovascular accidents Rate of recovery and decrease in number of limitations vary with each individual

Extent of the deficit for engagement in self-care due to the stroke varies for individuals.

Components of Nursing Agency

Theoretical Knowledge

Same as for Stage III plus

More in-depth knowledge of rehabilitation modalities for various types of neurologic deficits

Patterns of adaptation to long-term illness and disability

Skills

Same as for Stage III plus

More specific technical skill in implementing nursing rehabilitation modalities

Adaptation of helping techniques to enhance self-care agency and other forms of agency

Interpersonal style, which promotes healthful adaptation to long-term illness and disability

Ability to set realistic short-term goals and work for limited results

Ability to work with patient and family re: planning for future life-style and adapting self-care system to residual neurologic deficits

Ability to assume team member or colleague role on rehabilitation team

Stage V Health Maintenance, Continuing Care Stage of Cerebrovascular Accident

Population. Individuals whose functional abilities have been brought to an optimal level following a stroke

Health Care Goals

Secondary Prevention

Primary Prevention ⟷ Tertiary Prevention

Components of the Therapeutic Self-Care Demand

Types of Self-Care Limitations

Monitoring self for changes in health state, functional ability

Persistence of any combination of limitations identified in Stage III; each individual will have a unique quantitative and qualitative pattern of residual limitations

Continuing prescribed thera-peutic regimen (e.g., exer-cise, medications)

Persistence of excessive depen-dency

Seeking regular, periodic pro-fessional health assessment and care

Resumption of life-style asso-ciated with high risk for another stroke

Resuming system of daily living and of self-care with necessary adaptations

Pattern of seeking only episodic health assessment and care

Resuming social roles and rela-tionships in family and com-munity (or develop new ones)

Extent of deficit for engagement in self-care due to stroke varies for individuals.

Components of Nursing Agency

Theoretical Knowledge

Same as for Stage I plus

Common postcerebrovascular deficits and rehabilitative modalities

Rationale and expected effects of continuing treatment regimen

Family interaction theory

Skills

Ability to monitor health status with use of history-taking and physical examination and to detect signs of functional deteriora-tion or impending recurrence of stroke

Home, family, community assessment
Use of community resources; making of referrals
Health counseling techniques for individuals and small groups
Basic family therapy techniques
Ability to develop trusting, long-term, supportive relationship and
    to be client advocate
Ability to assume colleague role with other professionals involved in
    continuing care
Ability to monitor adaptations of self-care system for effectiveness
    and to help client re-adapt it as necessary

Nursing Systems and Nursing Roles   The structuring of
knowledge around the nursing systems variables according to
the time profile for cerebrovascular accidents contributes to
the identification of the ranges over which the patient variables can vary and the range over which the nurse variable
should vary. The *relation* between the *two patient variables*
during each of the stages of stroke was expressed in terms of
presence and extent of *deficits* for engagement in self-care.
A deficit relationship between self-care agency and therapeutic self-care demand is the condition that legitimates the
exercise of nursing agency toward the formation of a nursing
system. As indicated in Figure 5-1, *nursing agency,* when considered as a variable in a nursing system, is interactive with
both patient variables of the technologic nursing system and
with the existent relation between them.

Two questions still needed answers. The first was: What
would be the form and goals of nursing systems to be produced by nurses for individual members of populations designated by the stages of cerebrovascular accidents in models
for Stages I through V? The second question was: Accepting
the division of labor in nursing practice resultant from the
availability of nurses with different kinds of preparation,
what would constitute a rational distribution of nurse roles
in nursing situations where persons in the five stages of stroke
are under nursing care? The formulation and expression of
answers to these questions were guided by Orem's categories
of nursing systems [1] and Cleland's proposal for the categorization of nursing roles and levels of specialization [2].

The following descriptions of types of nurses (adapted from Cleland [2]) will aid in understanding the formulated nursing roles expressed in Table 9-3.

General Nurse. A nurse with less than baccalaureate level of preparation who is accountable for daily assignments, often functional in nature, and whose range of tasks has a high level of predictability and may be done with accuracy and speed; works in structured settings for an eight-hour day.

Nurse Practitioner. A nurse with baccalaureate level of preparation who is accountable for a caseload of clients during their hospital stay, or on a continuing basis in an ambulatory setting; who has a wide scope of practice and range of cues used in decision-making; utilizes the nursing process in working with the client and family during the entire course of illness.

Nurse Specialist. A nurse who may have less than baccalaureate level preparation and who has mastered particular diagnostic or therapeutic procedures in a specific area of practice; who has a restricted area of practice and range of cues utilized in decision-making although the nurse's knowledge base in this specialized area is more extensive than that of the general nurse.

Nurse Clinician. A nurse with master's degree level of preparation who is a generalist but who may have an area of concentration. This nurse assumes an expanded role and utilizes a very broad range of cues in decision-making. Although a nurse may concentrate on caring for a specific type of client, the involvement is very broad in scope. Independent prescription of nursing care, sophisticated use of the nursing process, and colleagueship with other health professionals are characteristic of the nurse's practice.

Based on the values of the patient variables and the relations between them for each stage of stroke, goals of nursing were formulated for each stage. These goals are expressed in terms of (1) a self-care system that is related to some preventive health-care goal; (2) compensation for self-care deficits; (3) patient involvement in self-care; (4) overcoming self-care limitations and promotion of adequacy of self-care agency; and (5) maintaining or promoting the adequacy of self-care agency as related to the demand for self-care (therapeutic self-care demand). The nursing goals are expressed in Table 9-3 in relation to the type(s) of nursing system that would effect the desired interactiveness of the variables to achieve each expressed nursing goal.

Given the values of nursing agency expressed in the six models derived from the analysis of therapeutic self-care demand and self-care limitations and given the projections of nursing goals and nursing systems for each stage of stroke, projections about the types of nurses could be made. The projections suggest types of nurses who would have requisite powers of nursing agency for persons under nursing care during the six stages of stroke.

The patterns of knowledge and skill required for the roles associated with types of nurses in Table 9-3 need to be made more explicit in order to guide (1) the delivery of nursing to persons in various stages of stroke, and (2) educational program planning at all levels of nursing education.

Further analysis and research are needed to differentiate the elements of knowledge and skills (and also orientations of nurses) that would be indices of the adequacy of nursing agency in each of the six stages of stroke. For example, the nurse specialist would need to have depth of knowledge and skill in neurologic assessment and physical care requirements in the acute stage of stroke. The nurse clinician would need to have broad knowledge of these areas, and to have more depth in the knowledge and skills associated with crisis theory and intervention and the integration of a comprehensive, long-term focus in the nursing plan for the acute stage. In the convalescent stage, the general nurse would have a minimum level of knowledge necessary to carry out a prescribed nursing care plan for this population and well-developed skills commonly required in the day-to-day care of this population. The nurse practitioner would have a broad preparation similar to that of the nurse clinician and be able to be more comprehensive in approach, but would have less depth of preparation.

Table 9-3 Nursing Goals, Nursing Systems, and Nursing Roles Associated with the Provision of Nursing in Each of the Five Stages of Cerebrovascular Accidents

Stage	Goal Settings	Types of Nursing System and Goals	Nursing Roles
I. Being at Risk (variable time frame)	Community agencies Mobile screening units Health fairs Mass media	*Supportive-developmental* Goal: Adaptation of self-care system to reduce risk of stroke; referral of extremely high-risk individuals	*Nurse Clinician.* To design prevention programs in collaboration with community leaders and to provide leadership and staff development to other nurses involved in stroke prevention *Nurse Practitioners.* To implement individual and group teaching and counseling in community settings, manage screening programs and referral, and follow-up of high-risk persons *Nurse Specialists.* To assist in screening programs
II. Acute A. Unconscious phase (days to several weeks)	Intensive care unit	Initially, *wholly compensatory* Goal: To compensate for complete self-care deficit and prevent further physiologic damage	*Nurse Clinician.* To develop nursing protocols in collaboration with other health disciplines, be consultant to nurses involved in direct care, integrate comprehensive long-term focus into the nursing plan, provide support to family, and provide staff development

B. Returning consciousness (1–2 weeks)		Gradual shift to *partly compensatory* Goal: To allow client to begin to participate in self-care. As demands for physiologic monitoring decrease, demands for emotional-psychologic monitoring and intervention increase	*Nurse Specialists.* With a 1 : 2 or 1 : 3 nurse/patient ratio, to perform an extensive range of diagnostic and therapeutic measures supportive of both nursing and medical goals
III. Convalescent (several weeks to month)	General nursing unit	*Partly compensatory* Goal: To increase client's participation in self-care and his adaptation to changes in self	*Nurse Clinician.* To develop nursing protocols, deal with unusual client or family problems and complex referrals, and provide staff development *Nurse Practitioners.* To assume primary 24-hr responsibility for a caseload of 8–12 clients throughout stay on unit, to coordinate implementation of nursing system for each client by general nurses working each shift with adaptation to changing needs and responses of clients and families, and to coordinate nursing system with rehabilitative therapies *General Nurses.* Responsible for most of direct care during 8-hr shift; work from protocols developed by nurse clinician and under supervision of nurse practitioner

Table 9-3 (continued)

Stage	Goal Settings	Types of Nursing System and Goals	Nursing Roles
IV. Rehabilitation phase (3–6 months)	Rehabilitation unit	*Partly compensatory* Goal: To overcome self-care limitations to extent possible, and promote adequacy of self-care agency	*Nurse Clinician.* Generalist with specialty area in neurologic rehabilitation to develop nursing protocols in collaboration with other rehabilitative disciplines, to intervene in management of the unusual or difficult client and family problems, and to provide staff development

Nurse Practitioners. To assume 24-hr responsibility for caseload of clients, to supervise nurse specialists and coordinate the nursing system with other rehabilitative therapies, and to engage in collaborative discharge planning

Nurse Specialists. To be responsible for implementation of the nursing rehabilitative plan for assigned clients for an 8-hr shift |

| V. Health maintenance—continuing care
Indefinite time frame | Ambulatory care clinics
Community agencies
Client's home
Long-term care institutions (when needed) | *Supportive-developmental* (optimal)
OR
Partly compensatory
Goal: To maintain or promote existing status of self-care agency, to meet specific self-care requirements or to teach others (family, friends) to do so | *Nurse Clinician.* To develop health maintenance protocols in collaboration with other health disciplines involved in client's care and to be available to other nurses for supervision, consultation, and staff development

Nurse Practitioners. To assume primary responsibility for the health maintenance of client and coordinate nursing efforts with those of other professionals and agencies involved in client's continuing care. In institution, primary 24-hr responsibility for caseload of clients throughout stay

General Nurses. To provide most of the continuing nursing assistance on each 8-hr shift (if patient is institutionalized) |

Summary   This construction and analysis of nursing system variables as related to the stages of cerebrovascular accident is offered as a beginning attempt to organize existing knowledge about a specific patient population within a nursing framework. It suggests goals of nursing and the design of nursing systems for individual patients and the design of delivery systems for providing nursing to groups of individuals who are at risk for or who have sustained a cerebrovascular accident. Further development and refinement of the models can lead to the identification of fruitful areas for research and hypothesis testing.

The review of the literature from a number of disciplines with respect to the entity *cerebrovascular accidents* and the organization of extracted items of knowledge around the *nursing concepts* from the NDCG *theory of nursing system* suggests that (1) these nursing concepts are good subsumers, and (2) specific pathology, in this instance a neurologic deficit with its sequence of events and results, does condition, at points in time, the values of the patient variables — therapeutic self-care demand and self-care agency.

The basic conditioning factor, cerebrovascular accident or stroke, is known to be associated with chronologic age and changes that occur with the aging process. The common expectation is that a health-care or nursing population defined by the stages of stroke will be an adult population. The influence of the adult status of the individuals or groups under nursing care during the stages of stroke on technological and interpersonal nursing systems should be subjected to study [1, pp. 132–134].

An Example of Multiple, Interactive Conditioning Factors
The preceding example of the organization of nursing knowledge involved the conditioning effect of cerebrovascular accidents on the values of the nursing system variables. In this example of knowledge structuring for purposes of standard setting for nursing practice, five interactive factors conditioning patient variables of technological nursing systems were

investigated. The example is taken from a project[2] to design nursing systems for women with uterine myoma hospitalized to undergo hysterectomy.

Five Factors   The general factors recognized by the investigators as having a conditioning effect on the self-care agency or the therapeutic self-care demand of women hospitalized for myomata uteri were: gender and associated developmental state, health state, sociocultural orientation, and health-care system elements. The multiplicity of the factors as well as their interactiveness had nursing significance. Within the frame of reference of the project the specific factors were identified as follows:

1. Female anatomic structure
                        and
2. The uterine pathology, myomata uteri
                associated with
3. The medical treatment modality of surgical excision of the uterus
                as interactive with
4. The location of the female in the developmental cycle of life giving, life bearing, and mothering
                as interactive with
5. The sociocultural orientations of these females and their significant others

It was recognized that the frequency of occurrence of the specific pathology considered in the project as a basic conditioning factor was associated with both chronologic age and sociocultural orientation. Chronologic age with respect to knowledge structuring was viewed in its relation to female developmental state rather than as a factor in and of itself.

The work of identifying and structuring knowledge about the range of variation of the basic conditioning factors and their conditioning effects on self-care agency and the thera-

[2] This project was conducted by Sarah E. Allison, Joan E. Backscheider, and Mary B. Collins with consultation from Dorothea E. Orem and Joan Nettleton.

peutic self-care demand was done in subprojects.[3] These included the following:

1. The development of a working paper describing myomata uteri including (a) occurrence by age and race, (b) cellular pathology, (c) location of the tumors, (d) effects on urinary bladder and colon, (e) signs and symptoms and associated pathology, and (f) treatment. The development of this paper involved a survey of the authoritative literature in pathology and medicine.
2. The development of a model to make explicit the major factors and the intervening factors in the *gynecologist's focus* on *patients with myomata uteri*. Four dimensions of the gynecologist's focus were named. These were (a) health-care, (b) medical science, (c) patient as person and agent, and (d) health-care delivery.
3. The identification and description of the phases of the medical management of the condition.
   Note: Subprojects 2 and 3 involved cooperative functioning with a gynecologist.
4. The development of a model of woman to identify conditions, factors, events, and actions significant for nurses to use in guiding their interactions with patients and in nursing diagnosis.
5. The identification of the range of the conditioning effects of (a) uterine myoma and (b) surgical intervention on therapeutic self-care demand and on self-care agency.

The subprojects were developed on the assumption that in the hospital phase of health care for women with the condition myomata uteri, the health-care systems produced for patients would have a medical component (operational both prior to and during the stages of surgical treatment) and a nursing component. Each of these components would be articulated one with the other and with patients' ongoing systems of self-care. Organization and coordination of these care components or subsystems thus would affect both the effectiveness and efficiency of the health care systems produced.

Organizing Focuses for Health Care   As the project developed, focuses were developed for use in identifying and formulating

[3] No subproject was organized around sociocultural orientations. However, forms and values of this factor were identified during both the nonclinical and clinical phases of the project.

health care and nursing goals and courses of action to achieve them. Such goals and courses of action would be general, that is applicable to all patients and to all health workers producing health-care systems. The identified organizing focuses are developments of the five basic conditioning factors named as significant in the production of nursing systems for these patients.

Focuses included the following:

1. The life-giving, life-bearing, and mothering capacities and functioning of women under care. For example, the conditions of being pregnant or not pregnant; having or not having children; being in or beyond the period of childbearing; or the interests, desires, and concerns of these women about childbearing.
2. The pathology of the uterus and supporting structures including the form, location, extent, and effects of the pathology; the symptoms experienced by the woman; and the effect on her human functioning and personal life.
3. The associated functional pathology of the bladder and colon.
4. Surgery to excise the uterus as the treatment modality and the psychologic and psychosocial events associated with a woman's decision to undergo this type of surgery.
5. Identification of problems associated (a) with being female and (b) with actual and projected changes in the genital organs.

Nursing goals therefore would be formulated and expressed in relation to these health care focuses.

It was recognized that the majority of hospitalized persons were likely to be *adults* with *definable capabilities for self-care* some of which would *not be affected at all* and others *not permanently affected* by the uterine condition or its effects. Self-care agency would be made *inoperative* during the period of anesthesia required for surgery but operability would be restored with recovery. The deficit for engagement in self-care would be qualitatively and quantitatively complete during this period. Prior to surgery, patients may be weakened from blood loss, discomfort endured, or under stress from all that is entailed in their life situations with *resultant limitations of self-care agency*. Both prior to and subsequent to surgery, nurses must attend to the *adequacy* of the patients' developed powers of self-care agency as related to the therapeutic self-care demand. To do this, the individual patient's therapeutic self-care demand must be formulated by the attending nurse working in cooperation with the patient, and both must take into consideration the physician's diagnostic and therapeutic plan of care.

The therapeutic self-care demand as generalized for women having surgery for myomata uteri would need to be formulated in relation to both the presence and the effects of myomata uteri and the surgery; to a range of reactions to the existent or projected effects of the foregoing; and to a range of reactions to the decision to undergo surgery for removal of the uterus. This project clearly demonstrated that basic conditioning factors should be viewed by nurses in practice situations not as static entities but as dynamic interactive systems. The term *basic system* as described in Chapter 6 conveys an important consideration for nurses in practice.

Summary   The example of the organization of knowledge around the nursing variables during the stages of cerebrovascular accidents was more detailed than the example presented in this section. This example was included to illustrate differences in populations served by nurses.

From a nursing population perspective, all persons with myomata uteri are women; the pathology as well as its effects are circumscribed, except in instances of severe blood loss or severe stress. The majority are likely to be adults with developed and definable powers of self-care agency. The operability of self-care agency often is not affected by the pathology and its effects, and only temporarily affected by anesthesia. Hospitalization would be required for surgical treatment or in instances of great loss of blood.

When surgical therapy is elected, hospitalized individuals would require the full range of nursing systems [1] at various points during the course of hospitalization.

The nursing of patients having surgical treatment for myomata uteri involves the use of a variety of technologies. Some of these, such as technologies directed to maintenance of urine elimination, bowel functioning, and preoperative and postoperative care, can be developed through the organization of well-validated techniques. Others, such as the technologies related to promoting maintenance of, or change in, self-image following gynecologic surgery, especially hysterectomy, are more difficult to describe in valid documented forms that are translatable to an action system involving a number of nurses. At this stage of knowledge development, it may be necessary in nursing practice settings to designate individual nurses whose function in specific nursing situations would be to deal with this particular self-care need using a partly developed technology.

The differences as well as the similarities in the two populations described point to the value of the basic conditioning factors in providing points of articulation with the nursing system variables.

In each example, the basic conditioning factor investigated in terms of its effects on nursing system variables was a type of pathology within the broad factor of health state. Both examples make it clear that the nursing focus was on persons at risk for a specific pathology, with a specific pathology, or at risk for an extension of the pathology. The perspectives of their (1) therapeutic self-care and (2) limitations for engagement in self-care were derived from or associated with the pathology. Specific basic conditioning factors within *health state* such as stroke or myomata uteri, because of their identifiable effects on nursing variables, are aids in identifying and describing nursing populations. The basic conditioning factor of health state includes series of events that denote normality or abnormality of human functioning as well as the occurrence of normal and abnormal structures chemically or anatomically described — chemical elements and compounds; genes, cells, tissues, organs, organ systems; bodily parts and regions and bodily form. The *nursing meaning* of *normality or abnormality* of human structure and functioning is that which must be sought by nurses in practice settings. A way of explicating this meaning when health state is biologically described has been presented.

Goals and Types of Human Actions as Components of Therapeutic Self-Care Demand

In situations of nursing practice, the determination of the therapeutic self-care demands of persons under care is a major nursing responsibility. One NDCG member's (Crews) fulfillment of this responsibility within an ambulatory care clinic for persons taking the drug sodium warfarin resulted in the formalization of a way for nurses to formulate and express the component parts of the total self-care action demand on patients that were associated with the use of a specific technology.

Prior to the opening of the clinic and during the initial period of its operation the nurse ascertained what was generally known about sodium warfarin as a form of anticoagulant therapy, including its consequences as well as the level of knowledge and the attitudes of persons taking it. A review of the medical, pharmacologic, and nursing literature was undertaken. Physicians and nurses who had previous involvement with patients taking sodium warfarin were interviewed. Patients' charts were reviewed and patients were interviewed with an open-ended questionnaire.

Ambulatory clinic patients taking sodium warfarin were observed over a period of time, and the self-care demand on these patients and the effects of the therapy were subjects of discussion and analysis at a 1972 meeting of the NDCG.

A General Set of Self-Care Actions   One of the results of this NDCG analysis was the identification that the self-care requirement for participation in anticoagulant therapy as prescribed by the physician through the use of sodium warfarin (a health-deviation type requirement) involved persons under health care in the performance of specific courses of action. These actions arose from the nature of the drug used for therapeutic purposes and from the need for continuous individualized management of care to promote drug action and to prevent or control toxic reactions to the drug.

One result of the analysis of the self-care actions required of persons taking sodium warfarin was the conclusion that self-care actions required in the day-to-day use and management of this form of therapy could be classed as (1) adjustments in or additions to existent *Universal Self-Care Requirements* [1, pp. 21–28] or (2) requirements that could not be so classed. Table 9-4 presents the demand for self-care actions

Table 9-4   The Demands for Self-Care Action on Individuals Taking Sodium Warfarin*

Adjustments in Universal Self-Care Requirements	Other Actions

Adequate Intake of Water
  a. Maintain hydration
 	
Adequate Intake of Food
  b. Regulate diet to avoid foods that interfere with drug action, for example, dark greens, fish, cooked onions
 	
Prevention of Hazards
  c. Avoid ordinary hazards
  d. Use first aid measures for control of minor bleeding
 	
Being Normal
  e. Oral hygiene
  f. Acceptance and internalization of short- or long-term dependence upon therapeutic use of sodium warfarin
	Set One
	  a. Regulate dose and take drug as ordered by the physician and managed by the registered nurse
	  b. Obtain prothrombin time at prescribed intervals
	  c. Identify self as taker of drug to others as circumstances demand such identification
	  d. Avoid the taking of substances that interfere with the desired effects of the drug, for example, salicylates, mineral oil, alcohol, oral contraceptives
	  e. Report to nurse the receiving of prescriptions for or the taking of any new drugs that may interfere with the therapeutic effect of sodium warfarin
	
	Set Two
	  f. Monitor self for bleeding complications
	  g. Monitor self for signs and symptoms of fluid retention
	  h. Seek medical attention when health-state complications arise

The health deviation self-care requirement: Participation in anticoagulant therapy as described by the physician through the use of sodium warfarin.

on persons taking sodium warfarin as formulated and expressed in 1972. The types of self-care actions identified in Table 9-4 were referred to as a general set of self-care actions for persons on sodium warfarin.

In the ambulatory care clinic for patients taking sodium warfarin, the nurse identified that ordering self-care requirements and related actions in this manner facilitates the taking of both a group or clinic population perspective and an individual perspective. The formulated and expressed *general set of self-care actions* served to order nursing actions as well as patient actions and provided a basis for evaluation of care. The general set of actions also served as a stable conceptual schema to which could be articulated other bodies of structured knowledge that previously had lacked points for articulation in a nursing frame of reference.

The value of the use of the general set of self-care actions for persons on sodium warfarin (Table 9-4) by nurses in obtaining information about the self-care actions performed by individual patients is suggested by Table 9-5. This chart shows (1) information obtained from patients about what was or was not done or about interfering conditions in relation to (2) two demands on the patient to take a specific course of action, and to (3) the type of human capability or disposition or conditioning factor involved (see Fig. 8-2). The *action limitations* of patients in ambulatory care clinics have meaning for nurses in relation to their formulation of goals that nurses can and should help patients achieve through the production and management of nursing systems.

A Model of General Ideal Set   The work of NDCG members in analyzing information pertaining to a patient population on sodium warfarin suggested to Anger the possibility of abstracting, from the sets of self-care action for persons on sodium warfarin, the goals and the forms of the identified and validated self-care actions. The purpose of this was to project a model of a general set of actions that would be required whenever a specific "therapy" to regulate any actual

Table 9-5   Two Action Demands on Patients, Types of Limitations for Meeting the Action Demands, and Associated Capabilities, Dispositions, and Conditioning Factors

Action Demand on the Patient	Described Action Limitations	Capability, Disposition, or Conditioning Factors Associated with the Limitations
Identify self as taker of sodium warfarin to others when circumstances demand this identification	Forgets what to say, to whom, when	Memory
	Is too timid to speak or take action	Motivational and orientative dispositions
	Loses identification card	
	Is aphasic	Health state
Obtain prothrombin time at prescribed intervals	Too sick to come in	Health state
	Arm is sore from venipuncture	
	Forgets to come	Memory
	Can't read instructions	Knowing and doing capabilities
	Can't understand instructions	
	"If I die, I die"	Dispositions affecting goals sought
	Dreads venipuncture	
	Does not understand reason for frequency of test	Knowing and doing capabilities
	Loses calendar that schedules tests	
	Too busy	Orientative and motivational dispositions
	In hospital day before, did not want to return	
	On vacation	
	Lack of money	Resources

or potential departure from a desired state of health would need to be incorporated into self-care. A model of a *general ideal set of self-care actions* was formulated and expressed in Table 9-6 in the form of nine types of actions divided into four subsets.

The expressed general model became a mental tool, a conceptual construct, useful for working with varied populations of patients from the perspective of the component parts of the therapeutic self-care demand that would be common to the population. The construct was verified initially with a population of patients under care for diabetes. Since then, it has been employed with other patient groups for organizing a nursing approach to patients with specific diseases who have demands on them to participate in specific forms of therapy through self-care.

Table 9-6   General Ideal Set of Self-Care Actions

Subset	Type
A	1. "Own" a self with an objectively established structural and/or functional state
	2. "Own" a self with a need for the use of a particular technology
B	3. Perform the actions needed to make use of the technology and to move self to the structural or functional state possible by means of the technology
	4. Perform the actions necessary to keep self in the functional or structural state produced by the technology
	5. Refrain from actions that limit the achievement of results sought through the use of technology
	6. Take the actions needed to overcome undesirable responses that diminish therapeutic return
C	7. Monitor self for structural or functional attributes that indicate an undesirable static state of response to the technology
	8. Monitor self for structural or functional attributes that indicate an undesirable regressive response in the presence of the use of the technology
D	9. Control factors responsible for (or productive of) a regressive or static state response to the technology

The nine types of self-care action named in Table 9-6 are believed to represent the extent of the forms of action that persons will be required to take to render therapeutic care to self through the use of a specific technology to regulate health state. The four subsets represent differences in the form of the types of actions and thus subsume different types of action having the same general form.

The types of actions within the model of a general ideal set of self-care actions can function as the intervening variables in the process of nurses' construction of the therapeutic self-care demand on patients. This process is conditioned by knowledge of the technology(ies) being employed to bring about some change in a person's state of being. If ways of meeting the universal, developmental, and health-deviation type self-care requirements are conceived as technologies and adequately formulated, then the therapeutic self-care demand can be conceptualized as having components in the form of sets of self-care actions related to the use of specific technologies being used in meeting known requirements for self-care.

There is a need in nursing to formulate the common components of therapeutic self-care demands associated with the use of a range of medically prescribed technologies. There is as great a need to formulate demands associated with the use of health maintenance technologies, technologies for primary prevention, and technologies to promote human development. At this stage of organization of nursing knowledge, the model of a general ideal set of self-care actions can be used by nurses in formulating general guides toward determination of the self-care capabilities of patients for using a particular technology in meeting self-care requirements.

Summary   The process of formalization of the presented models proceeded (1) from a nurse's seeking and having antecedent knowledge of a medical technology and its therapeutic use; (2) to the nurse's identification of actions that patients can and should take to incorporate the therapy into their systems of self-care; (3) to formalization and categorization of these self-care actions and their validation in practice situations; (4) to acceptance of the set of self-care actions·as a standard for prescribing and evaluating self-care actions for persons participating in one form of therapy; (5) to abstraction of goals and forms of action from the specific set; and (6) to the formulation, expression, and verification of a general ideal set of actions that would be invariant for the incorporation of any prescribed and formulated technology into a self-care system in order to meet specific self-care requirements.

The process described and the examples given make clear that the organization of available knowledge in forms useful for nurses in practice is dependent upon the work of *practitioners* who are willing and able to function as *scholars, developers,* and *theorists.*

NURSING KNOWLEDGE AND UNDERGRADUATE NURSING EDUCATION

An undergraduate nursing student is a person formally engaged within a college or university in learning how to provide nursing to individuals, families, and communities and in developing the capability to think nursing; at the same time the person should be advancing self as a nursing scholar and as a scholar in one or more nursing-related disciplines. The complexity of this educative process should be understood by those who teach nursing and design undergraduate nursing curricula. The types and amounts of antecedent knowledge to be included in a curriculum, as well as the form of this knowledge and its placement in relation to student experiences in nursing practice situations, continue to be problems to the curriculum designer.

Antecedent Nursing Knowledge in Undergraduate Curricula

Ideally at the level of professionally qualifying education in the university, nursing students would be introduced to nursing as a practice discipline with attention to the characteristics of theoretical nursing, practical nursing, and applied nursing science, including the nature of nursing phenomena and the methods of derivation of nursing knowledge. The stages of and the state of development of nursing sciences would be made clear to students. An additional focus on unanswered questions in nursing would provide students with a basis for understanding the need in the nursing community for nurse theorists, researchers, and developers.

Minimally, initial university education for professional nursing should contribute to the students' psychologic structuring of a body of nursing knowledge that includes:

1. The qualitative and quantitative properties of entities that are admitted into nursing by reason of a validating conceptual framework descriptive of what nursing is (i.e., a general concept of nursing).
2. The ranges of variance of the qualitative and quantitative properties of nursing phenomena and the nature of factors that affect the position of those properties at some point on these ranges.
3. Valid and reliable techniques for the control of specific nursing phenomena to bring them to, or maintain them at, a value or within some range of values.
4. Factors that will condition the effects of these techniques and must be controlled or taken into account as each technique is used.
5. Results that can be achieved from the use of specific techniques for the control of nursing phenomena and the relation of these results to human values, including life, justice, personal freedom, and states of health and well-being.

Structured, reliable, nursing knowledge in the above-described forms is viewed as essential if nurses are to move from a purely common-sense approach to problems of nursing practice to professional-level practice and at the same time provide themselves with a nursing base for research and development.

In technical nursing education the nursing emphasis would be on the kinds of nursing knowledge described in Items 3 and 4 just listed. The use of techniques in some types of nursing situations should be another focus. The types of nursing situations selected for inclusion in a program of technical education in turn define the need for knowledge described in Items 1, 2, and 5.

It is suggested that solutions to some of the problems of both the technical and professional forms of nursing education are totally dependent on basic agreements or the assumption of one or more positions about the characteristics and the forms of structured nursing knowledge. Both types of programs, professional and technical, should provide nursing students with the benefits derived from teaching and learning focused on nursing as a discipline — a structured body of knowledge that has reliability and validity. Rote learning and the development of habitual adaptive behaviors in and of themselves are in no sense preparatory for nursing practice in the contemporary world, though each has a limited role in professionally and technically qualifying education for nursing.

The designing of undergraduate nursing curricula and the teaching of nursing can be facilitated by involved nurses' acceptance of nursing as a discipline of knowledge and a discipline of practice. This carries with it the associated burden of contributing to the structuring of nursing knowledge through the development of nursing sciences.

Parker and Rubin [3] indicate that the function of a discipline rests primarily in its unique way of looking at phenomena, its modes of inquiry, its models for systematic thought, and its procedures for utilizing research. In practice disciplines such as nursing, there would be added the mastery of the investigative, prescriptive, and regulatory operations of nursing and the development of nursing prudence and nursing wisdom in making judgments and decisions in practice situations.

As previously indicated, the reluctance of teachers of nursing and curriculum designers to face the issue of structuring nursing knowledge in forms appropriate to practice disciplines in general and nursing in particular is a major deterrent to the growth and development of nursing in society. A major question in any undergraduate nursing program is the question of how antecedent nursing knowledge can and should be structured and located so that students can be helped to use it in obtaining empirical knowledge and in guiding their creative and doing actions in nursing practice situations.

The position taken by the NDCG is that nursing should be taught and studied as a practice discipline and that a *valid explanation of the reasons for relationships among nurses and their legitimate patients in a society* (a general theory of nursing) is the foundational and organizing principle for the practice discipline, nursing. Failure to take this position may account in part for the presence in nursing of persons who are willing *to do* but reluctant *to become and be knowing* about what they do and why they do it.

On the basis of the work done by Orem and other NDCG members to formulate and express the kinds of nursing knowledge usually included in undergraduate nursing education programs, Table 9-7 is offered as a summary of nursing content. The experience of NDCG members and the literature of nursing education reveal that until the late 1950s only cursory consideration was given to general nursing knowledge invariant in all nursing practice situations.

The types of nursing knowledge indicated in Table 9-7 constitute cores or centers for the continuing organization and validation of knowledge for practice purposes. The nursing concepts and models presented in foregoing chapters and sections of this book can be located in relation to the five named types of nursing knowledge.

The five cores of nursing knowledge presupposed for engagement in nursing practice provide the essential points of articulation with points of theory from nursing-related fields of knowledge. The development of each of the five cores of knowledge also would provide the points for organization and continuing development of *nursing ethics* and *nursing jurisprudence.*

The Roles of Nursing Students in Undergraduate Nursing Education

Nursing students are the persons directly served by programs of nursing education. Through them, both the nursing profession and the society are served. However, teachers of nursing are viewed as the prime elements in situations of nursing education, for without them there could be no formal instructional systems involving nursing students. A concept of *instructional system* viewed as the end product that teachers

Table 9-7 Five Types of General Nursing Knowledge to Be Mastered by Nursing Students

Factual Information	Nursing Knowledge Highly Invariant in Practice Situations	Nursing Knowledge with Lesser Degrees of Invariance in Practice Situations

Facts about specific populations in a society that can be helped through nursing	General nursing knowledge invariant in *all* nursing practice situations
	
	Nursing knowledge invariant when a nurse's patient is
	  An individual
	    adult
	    nonadult
	  A family
	  A community
		Nursing knowledge invariant in nursing practice situations where *patient* or *nurse variables* are conditioned by *specific* factors
		
		Nursing knowledge invariant in nursing practice situations where *specific, valid modes of helping* (or combinations thereof) have demonstrated reliability

design and create in cooperative relations with students was expressed by two NDCG members (Anger and Orem) who were involved in a project for curriculum study and revision in a university school of nursing. The concept has demonstrated utility for teachers and for curriculum designers and evaluators.

Instructional System   The concept, instructional system, as initially expressed was constituted from five interactive elements. Two elements are *person elements,* namely, *teacher* and *student.* Two elements are *knowledge elements — content* and *sequence of content.* The fifth element is *methodology.* Instructional systems were visualized as being generated within the context of an educational program and a curriculum, which set boundaries on the content and sequence of content elements that in turn imply boundaries for methods of instruction. Other identified constraints on instructional systems flowed from the boundaries imposed by institutional practices related to the admission to the educational program and to instructional systems of some students and some teachers.

Students as elements of instructional systems were conceptualized as having a baseline of physical and intellectual capabilities. Given this baseline, the operation of students in instructional systems was conceptualized as dependent upon their *cognitive, motivational,* and *psychosocial states* at points in time. The relevant cognitive state (state of knowing) of students was conceptualized in terms of their psychologic structuring of both nursing and nonnursing knowledge; the kinds of inquiry in which students could engage with appropriate guidance; students' use of conceptual constructs for subsuming data and available knowledge; and the facility acquired by students in the correct use of the language of the disciplines. The specific value of each of the foregoing for an individual student at a specific time would describe the cognitive state of the student and define the *cognitive dimension* of a student's *learning readiness.*

Motivational states of students would characterize their readiness and willingness to involve themselves in study and inquiry; to train themselves in mastering techniques and perfecting skills and habits; to be critical of their own advancement; and to seek help from teachers and opportunities for acquiring and using knowledge. *Psychosocial states* of students were viewed as revealed by their significant communications with teachers and others in instructional settings; by their formulated goals relative to achieving some status in the discipline, nursing; and by coordination of these goals with personal life goals.

Teachers were conceptualized as the main element of instructional systems. They can be characterized by their degree of mastery of knowledge and development of practice capabilities in two practice disciplines — nursing and education; by their knowledge of the curriculum; and by their empirical knowledge of students as person elements of real or projected instructional systems.

From an instructional system perspective, teachers are conceptualized as regulators with respect to guiding students' inputs for learning with awareness of the existent features of the cognitive, motivational, and psychosocial states of students. The teacher's function of regulating is operationalized through designing instructional systems that will enable students to (1) make required inputs for learning, and (2) regulate disturbances of internal or external origin that would move the cognitive, motivational, or psychosocial state of the student out of desired ranges. The teacher therefore affords students an active role in the instructional system and acts to facilitate their role performance.

Content and sequence of content as elements of instructional systems were conceptualized as varying with (1) the goals of the curriculum and the occupational form of the curriculum — professional, technical, or vocational-technical; and (2) the organization and prescribed use of the content of instruction in the curriculum design. The curriculum gives direction to the selection and sequencing of content by teachers and students in particular instructional systems. The curriculum serves this purpose through boundary setting for types and amount of content, organization of content, and sequencing of content; and through specification of educational results that the content, its organization, and sequencing should support. The selection and sequencing of content within instructional systems are guided on the one hand by students' states of learning readiness and on the other by the educational results sought by students and teachers.

Method as an element of an instructional system is conceptualized as a means of relating students to instructional material (that which needs to be learned). *Instructional material* is used to refer to all the sources and resources available to students in their endeavors to acquire and use knowledge in nursing practice settings. Method is adjusted to the achieved status of students with respect to the knowledge and practice aspects of nursing. Method serves to establish student and teacher roles and role relationships within instructional systems. Method should be selected in light of and be adapted to the state of learner readiness of students described in terms of cognitive, motivational, and psychosocial states.

Educators for decades have adhered to the belief that the five elements conceptualized as interactive within instructional systems are important to the achievement of educational outcomes. It seems reasonable to assume that together these elements may be viewed as a system of interactive variables; their type of interactiveness would be dependent upon as well as determined both by the nature of each interactive element and its internal structure and state in concrete situations at those times when there is a requirement for interaction of elements. Basic to the foregoing is the assumption that (1) an instructional system is a self-organizing system; and (2) teachers and students as person elements are selectors of and instrumental in the operation of the non-person elements, namely, content, sequence of content, and method.

The Student as Regulator   One ideal outcome of an educational system is that students as elements of these systems may come to act as perfect regulators to control disturbances that interfere with their achievement of educational results. The concept of the student as regulator within an instructional system context suggests that students function in two roles, the role of learner and the role of regulator of disturbances. As regulators, students would (1) know the existent conditions within self and environment that are related to the achievement of educational results; (2) become able to recognize and attend to a range of types of disturbances that would move conditions in self or environment outside the range that is compatible with their achievement of the desired educational outcomes; and (3) act to regulate, that is, transform, the disturbance so that educational outcomes will be those sought by virtue of studying within the range prescribed by a curriculum that has such educational outcomes as goals [4].

It is suggested that nursing students who have been introduced to and studied nursing as a practice discipline with a distinct domain and boundaries will be better *regulators of disturbances in instructional systems* than those who have not. Without such a cognitive orientation to nursing, students have no guidelines for sorting and organizing information and signals into those that are nursing significant and those that are not.

The demands on nursing students to function as regulators vary with the type of nursing instructional systems in operation. For the *five-interactive-element system* previously described it is suggested that instructional systems could be of three types:

1. *Teaching Systems.* In teaching systems the relations of teachers to students are clear-cut. The teacher has primary responsibility for
   a. Presentation of structured nursing knowledge and cues for learning
   b. Modeling to demonstrate aspects of nursing practice
   c. Active and direct supervision of students in practice situations or in laboratory type situations
   The role of students in teaching systems is primarily that of learner within a defined domain. The students' role of regulator would be limited by the defined domain of learning and the specific learning demand.

2. *Collaborative Systems.* This type of system is characterized by active mutual search on part of teachers and students for common insights as a basis for movement toward and exploration of pathways to new insights. The role of the teacher in a collaborative system is adjusted to the achieved status of the student(s) as a student of the practice discipline, nursing. Collaborative instructional systems may be spin-offs from teaching or self-instructional systems (see below); or they may be the system of choice in practice settings where students are developing the habits, skills, and the art of nursing. Collaborative instructional systems emphasize the teacher-student relationship as well as the roles of student as learner and regulator. These systems place high psychosocial demands on both teachers and students.

3. *Self-Instructional Systems.* This type of system emphasizes both the student role of learner and the student role of regulator.

   a. Students have primary responsibility for organizing and using instructional materials for acquiring and formulating nursing insights. Materials of instruction are teacher selected (regulatory function of teacher); adjunctive materials should be student selected.

   b. Students have primary responsibility for self-training in the development and perfection of skills — intellectual, observational, communication, linguistic, manipulative.

   c. Students have primary responsibility for identifying their own instructional requirements and for seeking out authentic means for meeting them.

   Self-instructional systems may be spin-offs from teaching or collaborative instructional systems; or they may be the system of choice when students are cognitively, motivationally, and psychosocially ready for guiding and regulating their learning endeavors.

Teachers as well as students must understand the *learning demand* placed on *students* within specific *instructional systems* as well as the *demand on students to regulate disturbances* in the instructional system. Since students function as elements of a number of instructional systems during a term or a semester, the control of the *total learning and regulatory demands* on students has been recognized by educators as a function of the curriculum and its administration. This form of control often is not operative in educational programs, and the need for it sometimes is supplanted by individual teachers who overwhelm students with learning demands that exceed their capacities. The need for cooperation and coordination of teacher efforts in the operationalization of a curriculum is self-evident.

The experiences of NDCG members in undergraduate nursing education support the discipline approach to curriculum design and development [5]. In relation to this, their experiences also support the need for insights on the part of teachers about the nature of practice disciplines and the characteristics and form of nursing as a practice discipline specified by a general theory of nursing. Teachers who are lacking such insights sometimes function as *distractors* to students within instructional systems, bringing about effects and results that are outside the desired range specified by the curriculum or outside the range that is desirable for students at prescribed points within a formal program of studies.

Values that can accrue from the use of a general concept of nursing and the conditions necessary for its use are summarized.

On the basis of the experiences of NDCG members in introducing and using a general concept of nursing in initial programs of nursing education, the following statements are made. One set of statements relates to the value of a general concept of nursing expressed in terms of the nursing students or teachers. The second set of statements focuses on factors affecting the use of a general concept of nursing.

Set One   The six statements that follow express values that can accrue to nursing students or teachers from the consistent and deliberate use of a reliable and valid concept of nursing.

1. The concept serves as a tool to organize current nursing knowledge from all areas.
2. The concept provides the boundaries within which methods of inquiry and thought systems are developed.
3. The concept serves as an intellectual tool to gain a nursing perspective regardless of the type of nursing situation.
4. The concept, as it becomes dynamic, enables the nursing student to enter into new and different nursing experiences with confidence when the new experiences are perceived as providing variation for an already developed theme.
5. A developed and dynamic general concept of nursing provides a career focus and assists nursing students in establishing an identity in the profession.

6. A developed and dynamic general concept of nursing enables nursing students to identify as nursing students in their relationships with patients, nurses, physicians, families, peers, teachers, and others.

Set Two   The five statements that follow express either conditions necessary for the effective use of a general concept of nursing or its utility in curriculum design.

1. Each member of a nursing faculty should have a dynamic general concept of nursing and the ability to make this concept clear to others in curriculum deliberations and in teaching.
2. General concepts of nursing used by teachers should not be so divergent that unity of curriculum design and consistency in learning experiences become impossible to maintain.
3. A general concept of nursing should be deliberately and consistently used in making curriculum decisions.
4. The elements of a general concept of nursing serve as organizing principles for the parts of the nursing component of the curriculum and in relating basic and foundational sciences to nursing.
5. The elements of a general concept of nursing (a) give direction to the selection and structuring of nursing content, (b) guide in the identification of context, which is foundational to nursing content, and (c) give direction to the formulation of learning objectives that have content and process components.

THE PRACTITIONER'S SELECTION AND USE OF NURSING KNOWLEDGE

The nurse practitioner's knowing of nursing ideally is in a continuous process of development and redevelopment. Development and redevelopment result from learning, which occurs in concrete situations of practice, and from systematic study of the authoritative scientific literature in nursing and nursing-related fields. The scientific literature available to and used by nursing practitioners determines in large part the rate at which they can advance their levels of effectiveness in nursing practice.

Nurse practitioners should be guided by the rule that *there is no substitute for empirical knowledge adequate in both quality and quantity for judgment and decision-making in nursing practice situations.* Generalizations, whether in the form of laws, theories, classifications, technologies, and so on, can only serve as guides in acquiring and organizing and attaching meaning to the concrete and particular and changing conditions of nursing practice situations. Antecedent nursing knowledge is used by nurses in their search for answers to the practice questions *What is? What can be?* and *What should be?* and in guiding their *designing of nursing systems* and in *bringing nursing systems into operation and in regulating their operations.*

Knowing, verbalizing, or attributing generalizations is never a substitute for having requisite empirical knowledge of nursing practice situations. This is illustrated by a nurse in a psychiatric setting who, in observing the abnormal gait of a patient with no history of difficulty in walking, *thought* "attention-seeking behavior" (inappropriate use of general knowledge) but, upon questioning, learned that the patient was protecting a "boil" from the irritation produced by walking (empirical knowledge).[4] General nursing knowledge is for *use* to guide the practical endeavors of nurses. Nurses *must have* and *must be able to use* and *actually use* both antecedent and empirical knowledge in the production of effective systems of nursing.

General knowledge, whether it be in nursing or in a nursing-related field, can be used appropriately or inappropriately by nursing practitioners and nursing students. An example of appropriate use follows.

A graduate student was meeting with a group of persons under health care in a psychiatric facility. A young man who had agreed to join the group came, stayed a few minutes, and said, "I have to go now." The nurse concurred and assured him he would be welcome, should he desire to return. In about ten minutes he returned again, sat down, then suddenly burst forth, "Do I look like a burned out schizophrenic to you?" "No," responded the nurse. "You look like a young blond, blue-eyed, good-looking man to me." The young man paused, turned, and asked others in the group what he looked like to them. Responses were descriptive of how he looked.

In the example given, the nurse demonstrated responsiveness to the young man as a *person* with responsibility for his

[4]Described by Cora S. Balmat.

decisions and actions (*agent* view) affording the young man the freedom that is required for decision-making.[4]

In the described situation, the nurse also followed the rule that in practice situations *questions asked are answered genuinely, honestly, and with a warmth that is nonpossessive.* In the instance cited, the actions of the nurse and other members of the group are presumed to have affected the young man. He became an active group member, interacted with members outside group sessions, and made the decision to get "his head straight" so that he could get out of the hospital (activation of powers of human agency including self-care agency). The nurse could hypothesize that the qualitative and quantitative changes in the *young man's actions* were associated with *changes in his self-concept.* And already-formulated theories of the relation between interpersonal actions and self-concept could be utilized by the nurse to aid in selecting or rejecting particular courses of action in similar practice settings.

In undergraduate nursing education, nursing students should be introduced to and master general knowledge in nursing and nursing-related fields that has established validity and reliability. The circumstances under which it will and will not serve the nurse in the provision of nursing care should be known by students. An example is the *constraints* arising from the *nature of teaching* on its selection and use by nurses as a mode of helping in particular situations of practice at points in time. A patient's inability to attend (because of extreme anxiety or other conditions or absence of interest) rules out teaching as a valid mode of helping. Such constraints are well documented in the literature of education and nursing. Yet, many nurses ignore or are not aware of them.

The selection of situations of nursing practice for instructional purposes in undergraduate nursing education should follow the rule that validated technologies of practice are formalized and expressed and have a known degree of reliability if used under specified conditions. However, students in programs that are technically oriented and in programs that provide the foundations for professional-level practice should be introduced to their roles in the more complex situations that they will encounter in nursing practice.

Nurses who aspire to function as the *professionals* who bear responsibility for the *entire extent* of the problem of providing nursing to specific individuals, families, or communities must be introduced to increasingly complex problems of nursing practice, including problems in which the general knowledge to give specific directions to practice is untested and may not be expressed in a formalized, integrated fashion. It should be unquestioned by a society that nursing students and young nurses who aspire to bear this level of responsibility in the society should be provided with practice opportunities under the direction of professional nurses who are masters of nursing practice in a range of complex situations of practice. However, this matter continues to be unaddressed in many communities and by organizations of nurses.

Nurses who aspire to bear responsibility for keeping selected dynamic systems of operations ongoing within nursing systems aspire to function at the level of technologists or at the level of technicians. They do not seek to prepare themselves to bear nursing responsibility to diagnose the "whole nursing problem situation" or to design the "total dynamic nursing system." These nurses do aspire to "regulate operations toward achievement of specific results." Nurses with these career aspirations and with education to support these aspirations have had thrust upon them high professional-level nursing responsibility. Again, nurse organizations and the public have failed to bear responsibility for the protection of both nurses and those served by nurses.

The continued attention of nurses to forms of nursing education without comparable attention to the institutionalization of nursing roles that are congruous with nurses' preparation demonstrates nurses' failure to view and understand nursing as a service and as a practice discipline.

CONCLUSION
The goals, the form, the placement, the sponsorship of education for the preparation of nurse practitioners have been

areas of dissent, frustration, and conflict from the first Nightingale-sponsored program to contemporary times. From the turn of the century efforts of nursing leaders in the U.S.A. to secure professionally qualifying education in university settings for practitioners have been thwarted by vested interests and other factors. Bullough and Bullough [6] point out that the difficulty in getting university recognition was due to several factors, including (1) the close relationship of nursing to medicine, (2) domination of the profession by women, and (3) preemption of the field of nursing education by hospital training schools.

Even more significant but related to the factors named is the lack of evidence that nurses consistently endeavored to advance and structure nursing knowledge as a basis for the improvement of nursing practice and education. This failure, no doubt, may be attributed at least in part to the third factor cited from Bullough and Bullough on the basis that professionally qualifying education broadly based in the arts, sciences, and humanities, and specifically focused on nursing as a practice discipline, is a first step in insuring the presence in a society of nurses who can conceptualize and theorize in order to understand nursing as it is, should be, and can become. A view of the whole of nursing, concern for its various essential aspects, and competency in one or more of these aspects are marks of the leader in nursing. The problems of nursing in the contemporary world seem to be increasing in complexity but the demand that the leaders see the whole (at least in its broad dimensions) remains.

Structured nursing knowledge based on a general concept of what nursing is provides some essential insights for exploring and grasping the dimensions of the need, and the demand, for nursing in the contemporary world. A series of questions is proposed as a guide toward the more rapid formalization of nursing knowledge.

1. What reasons validate the *work of the nurse in society?*
2. What generalizations about nursing have sufficient reliability and validity to serve nurses and nursing students in *real-world nursing situations* in collecting, grasping the nursing meaning of, and organizing data within the boundaries of a nursing focus?

3. What questions in the *field of health care and service* are properly nursing questions? What are valid methodologies for seeking answers to them?

4. Is available nursing and nursing-related *knowledge organized in relation to real-world nursing phenomena and questions of practice?* Are the *methods of derivation* of the various kinds of *knowledge* set forth? Is available *knowledge collated and readily accessible* or is it scattered? If it is scattered, how can this condition be changed? *Who can do* and *is willing to do* the necessary work?

5. What *stimulus situations* in the *real world of nursing* should be selected and organized into educational experiences at the various levels at which nursing education is offered?

6. What *technologies* and *rules of nursing practice* have the degree of reliability and validity that permit their inclusion in initial programs of nursing education?

The answers to the questions are viewed as essential for the continued existence, future development, and strength of nursing in our society. The work of answering the questions should not be deferred to future generations of nurses.

REFERENCES

1. Orem, D. E. *Nursing: Concepts of Practice.* New York: McGraw-Hill, 1971. Pp. 77–80.

2. Cleland, V. Nurse Clinicians and Nurse Specialists: An Overview. In *Three Challenges to the Nursing Profession: Selected Papers from the 1972 ANA Convention.* New York: American Nurses' Association, 1972.

3. Parker, J. C., and Rubin, L. J. *Process as Content: Curriculum Design and the Application of Knowledge.* Chicago: Rand McNally, 1966. Pp. 1–2.

4. Ashby, W. R. *An Introduction to Cybernetics.* London: Chapman & Hall and University Paperbacks, 1964. Pp. 209–215.

5. King, A. R., and Brownell, J. A. *The Curriculum and the Disciplines of Knowledge.* New York: Wiley, 1966.

6. Bullough, V. L., and Bullough, B. *The Emergence of Modern Nursing* (2nd ed.). New York: Macmillan, 1967. P. 170.

Index

Index